Table of Contents

Disclaimer

Nothing in this book, a collection of personal accounts, should be taken as medical advice. Always seek the advice of a qualified physician or health professional with any questions you may have regarding any medical concerns. I do not recommend or endorse any specific treatments, physicians, products, opinions, research, tests or other information mentioned in this book.

None of this information is intended to be a substitute for medical or psychiatric advice. Reliance on any information provided in this book except for entertainment purposes is solely at your own risk.

Other books by Amy B. Scher

This Is How I Save My Life

How To Meditate For Beginners

Lessons From Lyme Disease, Chronic Fatigue, and Fibromyalgia

Introduction

This book is a collection of stories, but more so, a collection of hearts poured out onto these pages. As the organizer of this project, reading through these stories has been bittersweet. The challenges of life are both heartbreaking, and at the same time, an absolute gift in many ways.

In a few cases, the story's author was experiencing an illness or condition other than Lyme disease, chronic fatigue, or fibromyalgia. These stories were also included because of their beautiful perspectives, and because, we are so much more than the disease that has been named and attached to us.

You will find that each story is written a little differently. Some are written as step-by-step offerings of how you can immediately apply another's lesson to your own experience. Some are written more as a shared journey, in which you will be able to glean whatever information calls to you. The lessons offered here are often contradictory to each other. Let this be perhaps the most important thing you learn; that we each have an opportunity to travel our own way.

When I almost lost my own life to Lyme disease and various health failures, I came to find my own truth. It is now what I share through my life, my writing, and my own work helping others heal.

"If treating the body alone doesn't resolve the challenge, then the body alone must not be what created it." – Me

In the end, all of the drastic medical treatments in the world were not my heroes. I was. My eventual ability to look honestly at myself and shift my emotions, beliefs, and energy that were a perfect match for dis-ease, literally brought me back not only to health, but to wholeness. I did this without blame or judgment (well, most of the time). I did it with a simple knowing that if I was part of the contribution to the problem, I was also part of the solution.

The emotional and spiritual healing work I did trumped the best medicine and doctors out there. It proved to me that while support may be essential, healing truly blossoms from within. As soon as I absorbed that truth deep down in my cells, everything changed.

Above all else, I learned a monumentally important lesson. Your path will unfold in its own time, revealing pieces of the puzzle only as they are ready to be healed. It will not always be in *your* time, but it *will* happen. The challenge is to show up, do the work, and peel away the layers. The rest will follow. All the while, you must learn to simply be in the flow of where you are, as resisting the process will drain too much of your precious energy.

There were so many people, places and things that I found on my search to 'get back to life' that I would never have encountered, if not for my sometimes-painful journey. It is clear to me now, you cannot just have the singular goal of *getting better* or you will miss part of what was intended for you.

Like one of my favorite gurus, Ram Dass, says, "You cannot rip away the caterpillarness. It all happens in an unfolding process...." I now understand without omission now what makes up the experiences of our lives. It is the energy of the Universe always trying to push us toward the light. It is the energy of our beings learning to flow freely, and without fear. It all works exactly like the wind, and although sometimes it blows in what seems like the wrong direction ... it will always come back to help us heal, if only we can just find a way to make ourselves ready. It is the biggest, most rewarding work of our lives.

This is how to follow a healing journey. You must become the ride. When you are, you transform all the parts of your being into strong, unwavering fragments of your whole self. You heal to your core. You finally realize that your illness was more than just years of suffering. It was the metamorphosis bringing you right back into all that you were always meant to be.

If we try to force the process of healing, we are not taking the full journey, which invariably includes why and how we manifested a disease or condition. This is how you make sure you never get back to that place.

Take what you resonate with from this book, and discard all that does not feel in alignment with you and where you are at this very moment. Be on your own path. Go your own way. Hold strong the intent to heal and trust it is coming to meet you halfway. Know you have more power than anyone ever permitted you to believe.

With blessings to you,

Amy B. Scher

P.S. To protect the privacy of the authors, personal contact information has been withheld. If you'd like to send a note to an author and there has not been a website provided, I am more than happy to pass it on. Please visit www.amybscher.com/contact to contact me directly.

Denise Springer

Chronic illness has given me far more than it has taken away. In all those years of suffering I never, ever, would have believed that it was easier for me to be sick than to be well. In fact, I would have had a huge ration of anger and rage toward you for saying it. Little would I have known that it was that very same anger and rage that was making me sicker.

Most of what made me sick was the false conclusions I drew from being restrained in a medical device at a preverbal age. My family's situation made it impossible for them to attend to me in a consistently soothing, emotionally-connective way. I internalized a sense that there was something horribly wrong with my very soul. Why else would the close breast-fed connection I'd had with my mother have disappeared? I was smart and learned exactly what to do to get attention. I oriented my being around what got me praise and positive attention. I was great at school so I slipped into academics. When hormones hit, I began to drink in order to keep the feelings at bay. I drank my way through Stanford. Then I raged my way through two marriages. I wouldn't let anyone get too close to me lest they see all the awfulness I thought was inside. Little did I know that they were just feelings – feelings all fermented into rage from being locked up for so long.

At the commencement of the relationship that would become marriage number three, I got sick – just a little sick. My immune system began to attack my nervous system. I was one large nervous ... system, that's for sure! But I continued to work and function. I continued to push.

We got married and had a child right away. Here came another huge blessing in my life and yet his birth brought a major health crash. It took me two years to realize how sick I was; I was pushing myself so hard that I couldn't see it. I won't drag you through all the trials and tribulations of an erroneous diagnosis (MS), multiple diagnoses (Lyme disease, mold-related illness) and a diagnosis for my son, as well. I pushed myself so hard I dropped. And I still pushed myself to inhuman, inhumane levels. I ran on anxiety and fear. And that was the best I could do.

Some majorly wonderful doses of humility later, my life has changed so much for the better and chronic illness was my wake up call, my touchstone, my companion which would never leave me high and dry, would always be there to remind me that I was valuable and worth self-care. Without it, I would have gone on injuring myself and others.

Here are some tips gleaned from my healing process:

It's your journey.
You will have helpers along the way, but ultimately this is all about you – your experiences, your relationship with your body, your thoughts and your feelings. Consider your health practitioners to be advisory consultants; you're the decider. Listen to what people suggest, do some research, and see what sticks with you. Go with that. This helps hone your intuition which will serve you well. Work with people who

help you build that relationship with yourself.

It's about "working with."
Focus your energy on working with your body instead of working against disease. What we resist persists. Explore how your body feels when you are tense, angry, happy, or excited and watch how that moves and changes. Get to know your body really, really well. It will tell you what's healthful and what's not.

Try energy medicine.
I started with acupuncture just to protect my organs from all the medications I was asking my body to process. My acupuncturist described my body's energy system imbalances at each appointment. Over time, I learned what feeling in my body corresponded with each traditional Chinese medical description. This has helped tremendously as I've moved on to do-it-yourself Energy Medicine because I now know which system to address; I can feel it and I have a name for it.

Acceptance.
You don't have to accept illness in your life forever, but you do have to accept that it's here now. Your body is trying to talk to you. Work with that.

Put your oxygen mask on first.
If you have any dependents, be sure that you are prioritizing yourself. At the very least, spend more than 50% of your efforts on yourself. If you go down, everyone goes down with you, so take care of yourself.

Consider trauma, stress, and PTSD.
At the bottom of most illness is chronic stress. This causes our bodies to mobilize for a physical fight which never comes. Without a physical fight all those stress hormones create damage. When this happens repeatedly, bodily systems break down and allow bacteria and fungus to take up more than their fair share of space, creating further imbalance. Get some help with your chronic stress so that your body becomes a hospitable environment for all those probiotics you're putting in.

Nothing is 100%.
No treatment or approach works 100% of the time. Find what works for you. Sure, that means you'll try some approaches that don't work. Congratulations, you've eliminated another therapy from the list. You're that much closer to finding the solution that works for you.

It's ok to see the cup half-full.
At one point, I wondered if I was going to end up delusional with all this happiness and positive thinking. That's when I realized that both are true: the cup is half-full and it's half-empty. The million dollar question is: which perspective makes me healthier and happier? Study after study shows it's the half-full approach. It takes quite a bit of brain re-training to begin to see the cup as consistently half-full. Be gentle about this. It's totally at cross purposes to try to beat your brain into new habits or to criticize yourself when you have a negative thought. Keep at it. Brains are super malleable.

Try forgiveness.
Practicing mindfulness-based forgiveness meditation was
hugely important for me. For 45 minutes a day, I practiced
slowly and silently repeating: May I be forgiven. May I
forgive myself. May I forgive [person]. The key is to allow
whatever feelings come up to just be. Often I felt anger or
fear at forgiving a certain person in my life, but eventually
my brain unwound from its attachment to the story of how
I'd been harmed. And almost magically, feelings of love,
compassion and deep understanding began to take its place.
For free downloads of meditation instruction on forgiveness,
search for "forgiveness" at audiodharma.org.

Develop faith.
Cultivate a sense that all will be well, that your life is
unfolding just as it should and at exactly the right time. No,
you're not being punished by illness. You're just learning
something really, really big.

Walk the fine line.
There is a fine and dicey line between knowing that you have
a huge influence on your healing and making yourself
responsible for your illness. When I felt responsible, I
became paralyzed with blame. I could not do anything
constructive for my healing. Always make sure that the
perspective and thoughts you choose make you feel
empowered, but not blame-worthy.

Have great boundaries.
I think boundaries are key for healing. You won't find me
calling other people toxic, but I will minimize the time I

spend around people to whom my body responds negatively. I may not be ready for their wisdom or their suffering quite the way it's expressing now. That's okay. My job is to take care of me and my body. One of the hardest things I did was to take two years off from being in touch with my family of origin. It was a tough decision, especially because my parents are up in years and I was afraid of losing them. But my love and tenderness for myself won out. I needed to give myself a chance to create new patterns and I couldn't do that with regular contact. My parents just being themselves would trigger my body back to a traumatic state. Those two years of separation were so worthwhile. I am reconnected with my family and feel more love and appreciation for them than I ever have before.

Learn to use your right brain.
Make art, explore your dreams, learn about symbolism, draw or write with your left hand. Each of these activities will use your healing, spiritual, right brain. Search the internet for other ways to switch into your right brain. If you want to learn more, read "My Stroke of Insight" by Jill Bolte Taylor or watch her TED talk.

Denise Springer holds a bachelor's degree in Human Biology/Neuropsychology from Stanford University. She is an Intuitive Astrologer, Dream Interpreter, and Transformational Collage Artist. She inspires and guides clients into their intuitive, spiritual, happy, healing brain. www.denisespringer.com

Scott Forsgren

Imagine a life where you seemingly have it all. Imagine wanting for nothing more, except for the continuance of your already blessed life. Actually, I never really wished for that as I always took it for granted.

Now, imagine that almost overnight it is taken away. This is how it happened to me. It all began with what seemed like a viral infection, and in just a few short days had become a major illness which continued to baffle the best medicine had to offer for days, weeks, months, and even years. My life was changed forever.

Imagine the fear one feels when presented with the unknown. Imagine the isolation and the desperation that one might experience when being confronted with a serious, unknown illness that, at the time, felt as though it literally could have taken my life. Unfortunately, it does not take imagination to understand what this might feel like; for this had become what was left of my life.

Imagine a constant burning sensation throughout your entire body that is at times almost unbearable. My body burned like someone had poured acid on it. Beyond the physical pain, there was the emotional pain which was generated by the uncertainty of what had become my existence.

Imagine having a fever that lasts for over a year, all the while having doctors and others trying to convince you that it might be "normal". In your heart, you know that this is far from normal, but you find it impossible to convince anyone that it is a sign of something gone seriously awry.

Imagine that you no longer have to imagine what it is like to feel sick day in and day out. Suddenly, it becomes you. You become it. Nothing else matters except the quest to return to your previous life. In fact, this was a new life filled with fear as well as physical and emotional pain unlike anything I had experienced in the past.

I remember it all so vividly from head to toe. Odd tingling sensations often ran through my body. My vision was blurred more often than not. My ears were full of pressure and popped with every swallow.

Walking was a challenge due to the weak muscles in my legs. For several months, I could barely walk at all. Of course, that fueled my fears that I had a serious neurological disease. Simpler physical acts were also surprisingly difficult. Sitting in a chair proved challenging as my balance was off. I constantly felt as though I was falling to one side. No matter how much I propped myself up, the falling feeling never went away. I always felt as though I was going to roll off the bed and land on the floor.

Every muscle in my body was sore and every joint even sorer. I cannot count the nights that I cried myself to sleep due to the intense pain. It seemed to get worse as time went on, and I knew that the illness was progressing and the need for answers grew stronger and stronger each day. I would stare at my hands and feet, feel the pain, and wonder what it was that was causing it. It was undoubtedly the biggest mystery I would be faced with in my life, and I set my sights on solving it.

I had muscle twitches throughout my body. Eventually, almost every muscle in my body would at one time or another have these annoying little reminders that something was wrong.

My stomach was an entire set of problems and symptoms in and of itself. It hurt all the time. There was an intense burning that never seemed to end. If there was a list of GI symptoms that one could have, I certainly had almost all of them.

Imagine a motor-like, tapping sensation felt continuously in your arms, legs, and feet. 24 hours a day, I continued to feel this constant tapping sensation. Imagine that every doctor to whom you described this sensation looked at you with a blank stare as if to say they had no idea what was causing the problem; or if the problem was even real.

Imagine the day that you open a book which describes a "motor-like" sensation as a symptom of something called "Chronic Fatigue Syndrome" (CFS). Imagine you search the Internet to find information on CFS which states that, "*The illness varies greatly in its duration. A few recover after a year or two. More often, those who recover are more likely to do so from three to six years after onset. Others may recover after a decade or more. Yet for some, the illness seems to simply persist*". Great, so now I had a disease which had no known cause or origin, no known cure, and even worse, it could last for decades. Oh, the fear and desperation that I felt, and yet, I could think of nothing more than to continue the quest to research and figure out how to get myself out of this situation.

Imagine that one day you find out that the cause of your unexplained illness is actually "Lyme Disease" and all of its not-so-delicious trimmings. Imagine you find a doctor that specializes in your particular illness and becomes your biggest mentor and influence as you now have something tangible to work with. Imagine that you work hard over the next several years to make a comeback. It takes work, hard work. You struggle. You sacrifice. You listen, not only to your doctors, but to your own body and your inner-wisdom.

After eight years of being sick, I found Dr. Dietrich Klinghardt MD, PhD in Seattle, Washington (http://www.sophiahi.com/), to whom today I express infinite gratitude for having changed my life in so many ways. It was his "Klinghardt Axiom" that became the blueprint for my recovery. It was the understanding that getting well is about much more than killing infections and that the infections themselves are often not always even the most important thing to address. It was learning about toxicity and how toxins are a significant factor in why we become ill in the first place. All of this occurs within the backdrop of the emotional conflicts and traumas that we have experienced within our lifetime. The axiom is about the interrelationship between emotions, toxins, and infections and the importance of focusing on all of these simultaneously to truly regain health and wellness.

Dr. Klinghardt pushed me to think outside of normally accepted ideas. I had to consider a number of new concepts such as how living in an environment with toxic mold impacts health, how parasites affect us, how electromagnetic fields add further stress to our already weakened bodies, the impact of diet on inflammation and immune health, and how other factors such as underlying dental issues contribute to the imbalances that we perceive as illness. The next several years became a pattern of removing stressful items while adding numerous health-promoting ones to shift the balance back to my favor. It was not easy, but it was so worth it.

Imagine that little by little you improve. It takes time. In fact, at times, the improvement seems so slow that you almost don't notice that you are still improving, but you are. Imagine that one day, you don't think of yourself as having an illness anymore.

Imagine that you learn so much from the struggle and gain so many unexpected gifts along the way that you never again look at life in the same way. Imagine that you create new friendships that are more meaningful than any you have experienced in the past. Imagine that you move forward in life with a newfound perspective and additional wisdom. Imagine that life is good and you feel at peace….at last you feel peace. Imagine, you are well.

Now, this was at one time hard for me to imagine, but fortunately, it did not take imagination because this became my reality. In my wildest imagination, I could not have believed that I would ever have gotten back to the place that I am today. I am truly blessed and forever grateful. Hope abounds...

Scott Forsgren is the editor and founder of BetterHealthGuy.com where he shares his 17- year journey through chronic Lyme disease. Throughout his journey to wellness, some of his favorite tools included herbal antimicrobials, detoxification support, essential oils, ozone therapy, photon therapy, and a variety of approaches to improving emotional health. He stresses the importance of working on microbial burden, toxic burden, and emotional burden simultaneously in order to regain optimal health. www.betterhealthguy.com

Jody Wilkinson

I am a 45-year-old survivor of Chronic Lyme and Chronic Fatigue Syndrome. This is the story of how I regained my health through understanding these three things:

1. Misery loves company
2. Ignorance is bliss
3. This is a marathon - not a sprint.

I, like many, had health issues for years before landing a proper diagnosis. From the time I was sixteen to my early 30's, I had a series of strange health issues. I was diagnosed with Viral Arthritis in High School, which knocked me off the Field Hockey team for several weeks. I was diagnosed with Cytomegalovirus (CMV) at 18, just after I had moved out on my own and dragged myself to my two jobs while recovering for about six weeks. Then after that, into my 30's, I would get mysteriously ill about every five years. My primary symptom was extreme fatigue and I would spend up to 20 hours in bed each day for weeks. Each doctor I saw called it something different.

Mono (misdiagnosed), Rheumatoid Arthritis (misdiagnosed), Epstein Barr Virus, Depression and eventually Chronic Fatigue Syndrome were some of the illnesses I was told I had. Ugh, what was I going to do with the diagnosis of Chronic Fatigue Syndrome? There was, at the time, no treatment. It seamed like my doctors had just given up on me and frankly, so had I.

In 2006, at the age of 37, I became very ill. I was very fatigued, experiencing tremors and losing my hair. I began to have problems with word recall, and sometimes even whole sentences escaped me. This was terrifying and it happened in the middle of giving a presentation at work one day. I just stood there frozen, unable to speak, while senior members of the group were waiting for my answer and staring at me. I was terrified of what was happening to me, terrified to lose my job, but most of all terrified of having to find a new doctor and go through the diagnosis process again.

Long story short, I found a Lyme Literate Doctor who listened, he ran tests, referred me to alternative clinics for more tests - blood tests, hair tests, brain tests, tests, tests. But most of all, he listened (!) and it felt like he understood. When I admitted to smoking, drinking gallons of coffee a day and eating candy at every chance I had, he said "Of course you are, you have zero energy and patients with no energy often turn to those three items. I'm going to help you get better." I was diagnosed with Chronic Lyme disease and hypothyroidism. Okay, a diagnosis!

He gave me two phrases that stuck with me as I progressed on my journey. He said: "This is a marathon, not a sprint" and "We have to peel the onion", meaning as we treat this disease, we might discover new things over time. And boy did we ever! I started a detox regimen to get my body healthy before we could even start antibiotics for the Lyme. This involved major diet changes, supplements, as well as weekly IV treatments at the doctors' office. I saw some immediate improvements and started to do some research on

Lyme. After I started antibiotic therapy, during which I decided to take a three month leave of absence, I got worse. I was walking across the Berkeley campus one night with my boyfriend on our way to see John Cleese (of Monty Python fame) in his one man show. Suddenly, something was seriously wrong with my legs. It felt like I was walking through cement and I was barely pulling myself along. I sat for a moment, and not wanting to disappoint my boyfriend, made the effort with his arm to get to the show. I spent the entire show worrying, what was wrong? I was thinking "How ironic, I am seeing John Cleese of 'the Ministry of Silly Walks' fame and here I am not able to walk!" I somehow got home.

It appeared I'd moved too fast on the Antibiotics and my legs were affected by toxins in my system as a result of bug die-off. It took me six weeks to regain my gate and boy was it scary. I had to admit I was truly sick, sicker than I had been when I thought I was at my sickest. Knowing what I know now, I know that was a huge sign to slow down. But, at the time, I thought I better do some research...

One of the first things I did was buy a few books about Lyme disease. The first book I opened had a dedication in the front to someone who had died from Lyme disease. I remember feeling instantly sick to my stomach and throwing the book across the room. Was I going to die? No one mentioned dying! I took a few breaths and said to myself, I was not going to die, this is a marathon and I'm already feeling better.

The next thing I did was join a Lyme disease support group.

Support groups can be wonderful, but they just weren't my thing. I found that I felt worse after attending and would spend a few days in bed after each group. The last time I went to attend, I was sitting outside in the parking lot listening to the radio. A doctor at a university in Massachusetts was talking about her work with bacteria and how she was able to dye the bacteria with a substance that lit up when the bacteria communicated with each other. She would push Petri trays of bacteria close to each other and the bugs would light up as if they were greeting each other. Well, that was my sign to start my cars engine and head out of there! I didn't want my bugs talking to other people's bugs in the support group and getting any tips on how to make me feel worse! Of course, that may have not been what was "technically" happening, but I did realize early on that misery loves company, and I might be better off keeping to myself. Listening to other people's stories often put me into a place of fear, which was not conducive to my healing.

From then on, I learned to listen to *my* body and felt my way along. I always did my best, even on my bad days, to dress nicely for my doctor appointments. I put a smile on my face and my best foot forward. The last thing I was going to have was another "depression" diagnosis. This "fake it until you make it" attitude did wonders for my healing! I also followed my doctor's advice and kept my research to a minimum (ignorance is bliss) and trusted that my journey, my marathon, would wind its way past the most relevant therapies. I would intuitively be guided to where I needed to be. If a particular protocol did not resonate with me, I would avoid it completely, or with the doctor's advice start with half or even quarter doses to see how I reacted. I certainly had the attitude that I would try anything, but also proceeded with caution if I had a feeling it wasn't right for me. For example, I resisted IV antibiotics during my years of treatment. I tried just about every oral and injectable antibiotic, but knew on some level the IV wasn't for me. I felt I did not need them. I learned to hold medicine or supplements in my hands and listen to my body for a "yes" or a "no." I worked with Alternative treatment providers to help ease the journey such as acupuncture, Bioset, hydro colon therapy, and I even traveled to rural Brazil to see a healer called John of God. All of these treatments helped in some way and I wouldn't have known unless I tried. I quit taking antibiotics and continued on a supplement only treatment plan in 2008. This was considered remission for me. If I was taking less than ten pills a day, I considered this "maintenance." I have had a few flares since then, and know from my experience, who to turn to and how to listen to my body and get back on track. In 2009, I began practicing Reiki, an ancient Japanese healing method, on myself daily. In 2013, I began to work on others. I very much believe that integrating alternative healing methods into my daily routine has put me in the healthiest place of my life. Recently, I visited a medical intuitive who told me I was on a higher dimension than Lyme disease itself. I recently visited my first Lyme literate doctor, the one who listened. He told me that when he first met me, I was so sick, he didn't think I was going to make it. Wow ... It's really eye opening to look back and wonder, if I had known he felt that way and not followed my program with a positive attitude, if I would be here to talk about it. I'll never know. As far as I'm concerned, my path was always to be well.

My advice to someone starting on their journey is:

Go at your own pace.
I mean that with regards to treatment, as well as regard to research.

Listen to *your* body.
What works for others will not necessarily work for you. Follow your own path.

Be open to alternative therapy.
Your body knows how to heal itself, but sometimes needs a gentle nudge or reminder.

Be patient.
This is a marathon, not a sprint.

Be positive.
Wear your favorite outfit to the doctor, smile, laugh, live. Attitude IS EVERYTHING.

Do not become the disease.
You are an important and loved individual - do not let this illness define you!
You can DO IIIIIIIIIT!!!!

Jody Wilkinson is a survivor of Chronic Lyme Disease, and Chronic Fatigue Syndrome diagnosis. She is a part-time high tech consultant in Silicon Valley and is an alternative healer

who practices Reiki, Earth Energy Medicine and is a certified Medical Intuitive. Jody resides in San Jose, CA with her husband Tony, dog Buster Brown and cat Tommy Girl. She enjoys interior design, and hopes to train to be a professional designer to add to her current portfolio career.
www.jodyreiki.com

Daphna

My journey with Lyme disease, also known as Multi Systemic Infectious disease syndrome started when I was 28 years old; 15 years ago.   My husband and I had just followed our dream to move cross county to sunny California with our new little family.

Unfortunately, the carefree California dream of ours came to a screeching halt just four months after my second son was born. I woke up one morning with an unfamiliar feeling of being unable to move or bend any of my limbs due to incredible amounts of inflammation in my joints. It felt as if my entire body had seized up over night. I could no longer bend my arm enough to support my newborn's little head to nurse him. In what felt like a 12 hour period, my immune system had completely crashed.

Looking back now, I had a few warning signs that my health was declining prior to this life changing morning. Eighteen months earlier I started having bouts of foggy headedness, along with a sense of being disconnected from my surroundings. I read every health magazine I could get my hands on back then and I looked into alternative healing solutions for answers. Nothing I came across could explain what was happening to me in that 12-24 hour time period.

During the nine months of my pregnancy, I had periods of extreme anxiety that began and ended with no recognizable triggers. As I understand now, being a biophoton practitioner (using EAV, electro acupuncture according to Voll to listen to and correct imbalances in the meridians of the body) and a medical intuitive, the anxiety I had experienced had its root causes in much more than the external stresses from moving cross country, as would be shown later.

After I had given birth to my second son, the anxiety continued as well as a whole slew of new symptoms: postpartum depression, inflammation in my joints and brain, swollen lymph nodes, chronic fever, pounding headaches, relentless fatigue, food sensitivities, dizziness, stomach pain and light sensitivity. I went from being a fit, physically active, health conscious, organic eating, adventure seeking traveler and doting mother to being bed ridden, depressed and zombie like in what felt like the blink of an eye.

I no longer had enough energy to shower, let alone cook a meal for my family. My cognitive function became so impaired once I finally made it into the shower that I didn't have enough recall to remember if I had already washed my hair or not. This was a very dark, confusing, and isolating time for me. All of what I had known myself to be was suddenly stripped away and I was left with no more than a shell of my former self.

To make matters even worse, my husband didn't believe I was really ill. At one point he asked for my general practitioner's notes, and saw she had labeled me a hypochondriac. This of course made his false beliefs that my challenges were really all in my head, even stronger. I was on my own in so many ways and up against a monster that had no name, but took my life as I once knew it.

Many years later, I learned that I had embarked on a set of health challenges named by Dr. Richard Horowitz as Multi-Systemic Infectious disease syndrome. Unfortunately, too many people have also gone down a similar road, symptom wise. Looking back at those frightening times, I see the most challenging part being the lack of support and knowledge from my husband, family, friends and doctors. As many can attest to, 15 years ago we had very few Lyme literate doctors. I could write volumes about the pain, suffering, and isolation I experienced over those years, but that wouldn't help anyone see the light of hope at the end of the tunnel. Due to the healing path I eventually found, I can gratefully say I am living more often than not in a state of wellness, once again.

This physical, emotional and spiritual journey has been intense, but the payoff from never giving up (not for very long anyway) has been immeasurable. I can't imagine I would have grown on all levels nearly as much if I hadn't been pushed to my breaking point so often and for so long.

It would be arrogant and ignorant for me to say we are responsible for all that happens to us in our lifetime. No one can know for sure what the big picture looks like. Though I full heartedly believe that if we approach life in that way, taking full responsibility for our life as if we have chosen every moment of it, we are less likely to fall into the downward spiral of self-pity and victimhood.

Therefore, I choose to see every challenge presented to myself and my clients as an opportunity to learn and grow. I believe that our life experiences happen for a reason, even if we can't understand what those are right now. I find taking on this perspective is the most fundamentally empowering and healing approach one can take.

Another lesson I've received through living with chronic illness has been how to listen to my Higher Self and the Higher Self of others, by remaining quiet and paying attention. From developing this sense of deep listening, I also learned that there is no better knowing than the knowing one gets from accessing her own information. Through my studies at the Academy of Intuitive Medicine and practice, I've developed this deeper ability to gather information, which is often referred to as intuition. I have learned that listening or intuiting is an art and a skill that is rewarding beyond measure and which we all have the capacity to further develop.

I also learned on my journey back to health that we sometimes must let go of old dreams in order to make room for all the new ones. As cliché as that sounds, this lesson was huge for me as my marriage fell apart along with my state of health. Sometimes there is more space than we like between one dream and the next. We must learn to trust that things are happening for your highest and best good and keeps life moving forward.

Lastly, I learned that everything is energy. Every thought and every thing you touch, smell, and taste is energy. Every unwelcome bug, virus, parasite or disease process is energy. Fortunately, most energy can be neutralized, harmonized or

.ted into a vibration that can be in coherence with our own physiological system.

So, how did I get well? I'm unusual in the sense I never did long-term antibiotics. Intuitively, I've always known the prescribed path of months or years of antibiotics was not meant to be my path. What worked for me has been biophoton sessions and The Emotion Code. The biophoton device I use is called a Cherin and it supports one's body coming back into its natural state of health. I use The Emotion Code to clear out any additional blockages that exist in the mental/emotional body.

For me, my healing path has been to work with light, my own light (biophotons) and through that experience I learned that light is the ultimate harmonizer. This path has brought me into balance within my body, mind and spirit. Of course, I fall out of balance at times, but I have the tools now to support and find my way back to my natural state of being. I hope sharing my story helped remove a little of the hopelessness that so many people carry with chronic illness. There is hope and everyone deserves to be healthy.

Daphna received her Masters of Intuitive Medicine from the Academy of Intuitive Medicine in 2012. She received her certification as a biontologist from The Institute of Applied Biophoton Sciences in 2012. She has been working as an Emotion Code practitioner since 2013. Currently, Daphna is studying to be a Body Code practitioner as well. She has a lovely home office in San Carlos, California where she works with clients (including animals) with all types of

health and emotional challenges including Lyme disease and Multi-Systemic Infectious Disease syndrome.
www.biophotonsessions.com

Carol Fox

"There's no Lyme around here," my friend assured me after I'd just found an evil-looking black tick attached to my chest. We had been hiking the day before near where I live in Santa Cruz, CA. Even though I knew people who had Lyme; even though I had a darkly ominous feeling about this tick bite; and even though I didn't know this person very well, I believed him. But I saved the tick, so I could ask a doctor about it.

A red rash appeared around the tick bite, but when I saw the doctor two weeks later it was gone. This rash, I've since learned, is a sure sign of Lyme disease; but I knew nothing about it then. I almost forgot to ask him about the tick bite. When I did, he dismissed it and said, "There's no Lyme around here." And I believed him. I really had no idea what the consequences might be if he was wrong. I figured Lyme was an infection so if I got sick, I'd get antibiotics and get well. I had other things to worry about.

At the time, I was working long hours as an RN and still in grief recovery from the death of my son two years earlier. I'd also spent two months working on a political campaign the previous fall, and had become severely debilitated working long shifts and eating junk food. The grief, the campaign, and my stressful job had me in a severely depleted physical state, and my immune system was a wreck.

All in all, my body was set up for the 'perfect storm' of Lyme disease.

Six months after the tick bite, my wrists were terribly sore. At times I could barely turn a doorknob. By chance, I came across an article about Lyme disease that filled me with dread. The most common symptom of Lyme: joint pain. Not a week later, I happened to run into the woman on whose property I'd gotten the tick bite. "Of course there's Lyme around here!" she exclaimed. "I told your friend that! I've been treated for it twice myself!"

Thus began the most challenging health crisis of my life. I lost my job, my house, my savings, most of my friends, and seven years of my life to this devastating illness. And it all could have been avoided with a few weeks of antibiotics immediately after the tick bite.

I sought out an MD who was familiar with Lyme disease and when I tested positive for Lyme, he wanted to start IV antibiotics in the hope of staving off wide-spread multi-systemic infection. But my insurance would not cover the IV antibiotics so I had a choice: pay the $4,000+ a month for several months of IV antibiotics, or take my chances with oral antibiotics. Once again, I made the easier choice and went with the oral treatment.

I felt better right away while on the antibiotics. But, a few months later other symptoms emerged, including profound fatigue, heart palpitations and shortness of breath. My well-meaning doctor did not recognize these as symptoms of Lyme disease, so he ordered just about every heart and lung test there was in the hopes of finding some other diagnosis.

Almost two years went by, during which time I became so debilitated I had to go on state disability, and then take an early retirement when the disability ran out. When the tests ruled out everything else, I became convinced that Lyme was indeed causing all these symptoms, and I finally went to see a Lyme specialist.

The specialist ordered a barrage of tests for parasites, viruses, fungi, co-infections, heavy metals, and other conditions which, he said, must be treated if I wanted to heal from Lyme. I came to understand that chronic Lyme is rarely due to a single infection; every case looks different because every patient has a unique combination of infections and conditions that have overloaded the immune system and are flourishing in the presence of Lyme.

The recommended treatment plan was more complicated than anything I had ever encountered as a nurse. I couldn't even begin this complicated and expensive protocol until I got the rest of my life under control. But my life was unraveling faster than I could do anything about it as my savings were melting away.

I ended up buying and moving into a ratty little RV. It seemed like a good idea at the time, and a sympathetic friend let me park on her property. But I spent the winter in a cold, damp, cramped little box, feeling hopeless and, basically, homeless. In two years, I had gone from living in a beautiful home with a lucrative job and high hopes for retirement to living in this miserable RV on the last of my savings, unable to follow the protocol ordered by the specialist.

My illness had progressed to affecting my brain, and I couldn't focus or get organized, no matter how hard I tried. I later learned that this 'brain fog' is a common symptom and is caused by the build-up of Lyme toxins. At the time, I thought I was going crazy. I began to fear that I could actually die of this illness. I couldn't get it together, either cognitively or financially, to do what it was going to take to get better. And I was getting worse.

When all seemed hopeless, a family member learned of my illness, sent me a generous check and told me to get some help right away. Encouraged by her support, I made another appointment with the specialist, and with a Lyme-knowledgeable acupuncturist as well.

I started the first phase of treatments in what would be a four-year journey back from Lyme hell. With family help, I got out of the RV and into a rented room. I was making modest gains and starting to feel more functional. But my progress was painfully slow. Because of the expense and the complicated treatments, my 'compliance' was not the best; I still didn't understand the need for all the treatments and was not motivated to do all that needed to be done.

One afternoon I was lying on the acupuncturist's table with about 20 needles in me, feeling particularly discouraged and thoroughly victimized by this horrid disease that was ruining my life. And out of nowhere, a voice from deep inside me said, very loud and clear, "I am not going to let this take me down!" In that moment, everything shifted. It was as if I got up from the table a different person than the one who had been lying there. I looked the same and I was still very sick. I knew at this point that I was willing to go to any lengths to get better, and that it was just a matter of time; I was going to heal.

One of the first things I had to do was end a seven-year friendship that had become destructive to both of us. My friend readily agreed and seemed relieved to let it go. I mourned our friendship, but immediately felt empowered by the decision.

About that time I met another Lyme specialist, and I knew I had found the doctor who could help me get well. His treatment protocols were similar, but unlike my first doctor, this one was an empathetic, spiritual young man with an uplifting, positive attitude, and a firm belief that Lyme could be cured because he had healed himself.

He ordered more tests, more procedures, and more medications. But now, there were also explanations. I understood why it was all necessary, and with this understanding, I was able to cooperate much more fully. Now, I was willing to do whatever it would take. I was very fortunate that my family members were willing and able to help me with the finances. But if they had not, I was prepared to go into debt to get the treatment. I had wasted four years trying unsuccessfully to hang on to my money, meanwhile losing years of my life. Now, I had my priorities straight: health first, and figure out the finances later.

Recovery became my full-time job, and it was a lot of work. I was taking 35 different medications and supplements a day, plus daily aggressive detox procedures, and preparing all my meals from scratch to support my healing. Very gradually, I started to see some real improvement. And as I felt better, I was able to do more. Uplifting activities like Dance Church, art classes, and gardening were healing for my body and mind. I was starting to get some semblance of a life.

Further testing revealed that I was severely sensitive to mold and unfortunately my house was saturated with mold. As if by divine design, my housemate gave notice and my name came up on the waiting list for low-income housing in the same week. A month later, I was in my own little mold-free apartment and I soon was feeling loads better.

I continued on my Lyme program for several months, but after that move my recovery went relatively smoothly. A year later, using electronic testing, I tested negative for Lyme for the first time in seven years.

As happy as I was to be free of Lyme, I had to mourn as well. For seven years I had played the role of the Very Sick Person, afflicted with this mysterious illness that made me quite special and absolved me of many responsibilities. I was now back among the ordinary citizens of the world, somewhat weaker and seven years older, but not extraordinary anymore. It took me several weeks to process this loss, but of course in the long run I knew Lyme was a great thing to lose.

In the beginning, I had listened to everyone around me but not to my own brilliant, intuitive body, and the consequences could hardly have been more dire. In Lyme recovery, I have learned to listen to my own inner voice first and last; not ignoring input from others, but filtering it through what I have come to understand is my own best friend, ME.

I have learned that I am made of tougher stuff than I ever imagined – I am a Survivor. Prior to Lyme, I never knew I had the grit to face down such a foe and win. That voice I heard on the acupuncturist's table had to overcome a powerful program of victimhood and learned helplessness that would have taken me down.

I've learned not to get stuck in resentment or fear. In recovery, I had to let go of my resentment toward the doctors, friends, and family members who didn't believe I had Lyme. And I had to see each obstacle as an opportunity to change and grow, instead of letting problems stop me. I had to overcome my aversion to drugs, my confusion about the treatments, my dependent attitude that wanted somebody else to take care of me and make this illness go away.

I learned about the power of gratitude. Even when I was sick, I needed to find things to be grateful for – the kindness of a friend, the string beans growing in my garden, the kitty who kept me company when I was stuck in the house. Like many people who have gone through serious illness, I now have a deeper appreciation for every day I am alive and well. I have lost much, but gained much too, and am a better person for the experience.

Carol Fox is an RN, writer and artist. She has traveled unscathed throughout the US and Central America and had many hair-raising adventures before settling down in California to save for retirement, only to be brought to her knees by a tick the size of a sesame seed. She fought a 7-year battle with Lyme Disease and went through some very dark times, but in the process, found an inner strength she didn't know she had. She is now completely free of Lyme. She has created an entertaining and educational slide show (currently being made into a DVD, and a website is in progress) about how to avoid Lyme disease and teaches a class on the same topic. Carol lives with her dog, Bonnie, in Santa Cruz, CA.

www.theticklady.weebly.com

Reinhard

I was diagnosed with Lyme (Borrelia) via a direct blood culture test from Advanced Laboratory. The test showed color stained microbes. I am not sure how long the microbes had been in my body or how they got there.

I had never noticed a tick bite, but I had felt tired and sluggish for a couple of years before and I did have a weird fever earlier that summer. It was starting to affect me in my daily life. And just a couple weeks after the diagnosis, my joints and muscles actually started to hurt and typical Lyme symptoms started to kick in.

I knew right away what this meant. My wife had been diagnosed with Lyme three years earlier and I had watched her condition deteriorate and our time together was spent in our home – her activities were limited.

Because of my wife's condition, I had a head start going into the Lyme experience. I saw what worked and what didn't work for her and knew about the traditional, as well as alternative options for treatment based on my research.

What followed next was a rollercoaster of ups and downs - going through conventional and alternative treatments across two continents. Being from Europe, I was able to take time off and go back to my home town Vienna, Austria for alternative treatments not available in the US. While in the U.S., I was working with an excellent Lyme literate MD and an experienced Klinghardt trained kinesiology tester. Looking back now at the last year and a half of my healing, I was able to categorize the protocols I had put together for myself.

Antibiotics, IVs and antimicrobials.

I entered the treatment process based on the experiences of my former Austrian family MD who had good experience treating Lyme patients in his practice. He used IV antibiotics (conventional intracellular antibiotics) and combined them with Ozone Hemotherapy.

In addition to IV antibiotics that would go after the spirochete and L-form, I also took oral antibiotics that would kill the cyst form based on advice from my Lyme literate MD. I also took an oral intracellular antibiotic that worked well with the IVs. In total, I was on two to three antibiotics for a period of about seven months.

While on pharmaceutical IVs and antibiotics, I started to take natural antimicrobials in the form of essential plant oils. Plants naturally produce various antimicrobial substances to defend themselves against environmental threats such as fungus or bacteria. Taking the oils as capsules was essential as it allowed me to get off antibiotics sooner. Later on I added other herbal antimicrobials, mostly for support or to fight possible co-infections.

Ozone treatments.
Ozone (O3) is a gas, more potent than Oxygen, which creates massive oxidative stress for anaerobic organisms.

During Hemotherapy, about 250ml of blood is taken from the patient's body via IV and pumped into a glass bottle. The bottle is filled with ozone gas which is immediately absorbed by the blood and then the blood is dripped back into the body. Ozone works well with IV antibiotics as it creates an initial toxic environment for Borrelia. This allows antibiotics to better kill the weakened microbes. I later performed Ozone therapy at home by ozonating my drinking water.

Hyperthermia therapy.
As antibiotics and oxygen attack Borellia in the body, the bacteria may start to drill deeper into connective tissue or joints and become harder to reach. Increasing body temperature helps stimulate the body's own immune system to naturally fight those hard to reach Borellia. During a hyperthermia session the body is gradually, over a period of about four hours, heated up to a temperature of 103-104 degrees Farenheit while being hooked up to IVs. In some clinics, temperatures are being driven up to 107 degrees, but that is performed under anesthesia only.
I did 15 Hyperthermia sessions in Vienna over a period of one year and am planning to continue with one to two treatments per year for "maintenance" purposes.

In my experience, hyperthermia acts as an accelerator in curing Lyme. It activates the immune system, helps excrete toxins, and provides healing stimuli. After my hyperthermia treatments were completed, I continued home heat treatments with a small portable infrared sauna on a bi-weekly basis. As I got better and got my energy back, I added occasional Bikram Yoga to the heat practice.

Addressing biofilms.
It is known that Lyme bacteria are able to form biofilms along with other microorganisms making them hard to reach by antibiotics. I added biofilm breakers to my daily protocols from the beginning. These included biofilm enzymes, NAC, and EDTA to chelate metals or calcium out of the biofilms and grapefruit seed extract to create a "soapy" environment. Often, I followed the biofilm protocol with hyperthermia, ozone or infrared sauna sessions to create a "thorough hot wash" environment in my body, together with essential oils which would kill off any exposed bacteria.

Detoxification.
To help release die off toxicity from the body, I applied multiple detox protocols on a daily basis which included Chlorella or charcoal. I also worked with natural intestinal binders to stop re-absorption of toxins from gall fluid in the intestinal tract such as Guggul. And during critical times, I used glutathione IVs and high amounts of Vitamin C on a weekly basis to help with toxin release.

I also performed colonics and occasional liver cleanses (Moritz Liver Gallbladder flush) to keep everything clean. Even though I did all that cleansing work, I still developed liver and kidney problems after taking antibiotics for seven months and I am still working on getting those two organs fully back in shape. I believe constant detoxing is absolutely critical in the Lyme healing process and one can't do enough of it.

Emotional work and energy testing.

While I was going through my treatments I kept thinking that there had to be a reason why I got ill in the first place. I came across Dr. Klinghardt's Detoxification Axiom which helped me better understand what happened. Dr. Klinghard states that the amount of pathogenic organisms and toxins in the body go hand in hand with unresolved emotional trauma. All of those things had to be resolved simultaneously. It became clear to me that my emotional and energy body had to be addressed as well.

Whenever visiting Austria, I worked with a holopathic doctor who used meridian-energy based measurement techniques to determine organ status and microbial stress. He was able to identify emotional blockages, applied frequency based energy treatments, and tested the right essential oils treatments. I also worked with a reconnective therapy practitioner in the U.S. who helped facilitate the reconnection between the energy body and the physical body, thus allowing the release of stored patterns and a return to the original blueprint."

Just like measuring performance of a business, one needs to establish a closed loop system of periodic testing and treatment adjustments. Unfortunately, standard Lyme and co-infection testing is expensive and not well suited for ongoing performance evaluation. I decided to work with one of the best Klinghardt trained ART (Kinesiology) testers in the US to receive insights for microbial stressors, drugs, supplements and blocking conditions.

General system support.

While staying on my protocols, I added supplements for core system support. This included anti-inflammatories such as Curcumin, Japanese Knotweed, and MSM for muscle and joint pain. For basic energy and strength, I used Vitamin D, Vitamin B12/B Complex, CoQ10, L-Argentine and Siberian Ginseng. Based on hormonal panels, I also added hormonal support to improve sleep and energy. In addition, I added digestive and intestinal support and Candida fighters to keep my system as balanced as possible. To address heart palpitations, I used homeopathic Strophantus, as well Hawthorn extract.

I had already optimized my nutrition in prior years due to unrelated health issues and was on a high vegetable, low carb, no grain/gluten, mostly Paleo diet. When diagnosed with Lyme, I was generally fit and getting good nutrition, which was a big advantage.

Although I had very low energy at times, I tried to go on walks as often as possible. My eyes had become light sensitive and I felt that Borrelia wanted me to stay indoors. I literally tried to do the opposite, get as much oxygen as possible, avoid sunglasses, and move around in the sun as much as I could.

Good fortune and attitude.

I was very lucky to learn from the best people in the field and receive their help in my healing process. I was also fortunate to have the financial resources and the support in my professional environment, allowing me to spend time on treatments.

I believe personal attitude during the healing process is critical. I had my setbacks, and I still have them as I clear out toxins and deal with secondary infections. There were times when my veins burned after IVs, when old symptoms came back or new ones developed. Even while writing this book contribution, some old muscle pains are starting to flame up again. All in all, one has to be in this for the long haul and not get discouraged. What counts is the overall journey.

A final note.
When fighting Lyme, you have to use every resource at your disposal while keeping yourself as healthy as possible. Over time, Borrelia may attack the nervous system and impair cognitive function. This means there may be times when your thinking is fuzzy and harder for you. The focus of your life needs to shift fully towards "project managing" your healing process with the help of multiple professionals.

It is absolutely critical to understand that oral antibiotics alone will not get you healthy unless Lyme is caught very early on. This has been my experience. You need to address your illness on all levels, physically using conventional and alternative medicine and energetically and emotionally to regain your full health.

Reinhard is a mobile technology expert based in the Silicon Valley. Reinhard has always had a longing for deeper understanding beyond technology and has spent a great deal of time exploring fields such as spirituality, philosophy, cosmology as well as health, nutrition, and herbs. Reinhard has lived and worked on two continents and loves traveling, discovering new cultures, and exploring nature. He enjoys writing and has authored and published bestselling Internet handbooks in the German language. Reinhard has a MSEE in Telecommunications from Santa Clara University, CA and an engineering degree from the Technical University of Vienna.

www.lyme-treatment.com

Lisa

One week after I went to the OEC (Outdoor Education Center) with my daughter's third grade class in May of 2010, I was having knee pain and discovered a rash. I went into care, was told it was Lyme, and was given a prescription of Doxycycline. I started taking it as prescribed, thinking the pain would leave and I'd be good to go.

Yeah right! That did not happen.

Instead, more symptoms kicked in: ringing in my ears, chills, confusion, brain fog, crying, forgetfulness, mixing words/sounds up, weak muscles, profound fatigue, intense feelings of being overwhelmed/overstimulated, light and sound sensitivities, lots of muscle and joint pain and the list goes on.

A few months later, I hit lower lows and darkness than I ever have in my life. I called our 211 hotline (our local information and referral/crisis hotline, which is available in each state) and did counseling for a year.

I had a difficult time with the Lyme controversy and animosity between the two opposing sides. I became fearful of ticks and woodsy areas. I avoided them and had my family do the same.
All I could think about was "Lyme." I learned everything I could, kept track of my symptoms, joined groups and went to meetings.

I saw people with chronic Lyme, attached to IVs, who had been treating for months, years, and yet, they were still suffering. Some couldn't even walk they were so weak. Others were figuring out how to claim disability.

From the get-go, I was uncomfortable with the label "Lymie" that was given to me (with good intentions by people with big hearts) when I joined the support groups.

And I remember wanting so badly to talk with people who were getting better, who had overcome, who were filled with HOPE.

I saw four doctors, three massage therapists, two biofeedback practitioners, two chiropractors, two Reiki practitioners, two psychics, two therapists, two Native American healers, an acupuncturist, a spiritual director, a nutritionists (and a partridge in a pear tree).

After all that, I wasn't seeing much improvement in my symptoms.

After about two years, I STOPPED. I stopped reading about Lyme, treating, and doing the symptom journal. I was sick of it all and needed a break.

I eventually came upon Amy Scher's book, "This is How I Save My Life." I admired the way she put it all out there, amazed at what she went through...came through. I could relate to her feelings about emotional work being a missing piece of the puzzle. I got it!

Amy's story prompted me to start asking myself why I felt the need to tell people I had Lyme, how having Lyme might have served me: been a way to slow down, have an excuse to take a break, be cared for and for others to see I was hurting. I'm not sure exactly how Lyme was serving me, but those things crossed my mind.

I believe the symptoms were saying, "Hey, Lisa, what's going on here? Something's 'off.' I can show you the way if you let go of that control. Release what you're holding onto so tightly. I realize you are doing that to protect yourself, but it is okay…"

Looking back, I realize that much of what I was doing and taking in those first years was not helpful. I was looking outside myself for healing and I was filled to the brim with fear. An yet, it was what I needed to do to get to a better place.

I've come a long way in the four years since the Lyme diagnosis.

I'm no longer running away from my strong emotions. I'm honoring them, asking what they can teach me, and befriending the darkness.

I'm realizing that the Universe/Creator is kind and supportive, not hostile. And that at our core is goodness.

I understand others who struggle with darkness. I'm finding

my judgments being replaced with compassion. I feel a deep connection to others, to nature.

I realize that my husband is going to stick with me, even in the hard times. He did, and continues to. For that, and him, I am grateful.

I realize that I've always had, and always will have, within me—everything I need for healing.
To quote The Wizard of Oz:

Dorothy: Is there a way for me to get back home?

Glinda : You were wise and good enough to help your friends come here and find what was inside them all the time. That's true for you, also.

Dorothy: Home? Inside of me? I don't understand.

Glinda: Home is a place we all must find, child. It's not just a place where you eat or sleep. Home is knowing, knowing your mind, knowing your heart, knowing your courage. If we know ourselves, we're always home, anywhere.

Another silver lining on my Lyme journey is that I set myself free spiritually. While I honor my Lutheran and Catholic roots and all that my ancestors went through for religious freedom, I no longer need or want the label "Lutheran" or "Catholic" or anything else. My spirituality is strong. It doesn't matter what anyone else thinks about that. As the Dalai Lama said: "My religion is kindness." Any spiritual figure or ideas that support love, peace, and kindness are ones I'm open to.

I'm learning, thanks to Byron Katie, to question my thoughts, especially those creating suffering. "Don't believe everything you think."

I'm doing more to take care of myself. I have massages twice a month, yoga weekly. I'm finding time to be still, quiet.

An amazing positive of this journey is that I appreciate the people in my life more and am more often in-the-moment with them.

I'm also taking time to have fun, do things I love.

I'm keeping an eternal perspective.

Throughout my journey, I've been blessed with family who care and are there, providing love and support. One of my biggest supporters in this journey has been my sister. She helped me see things from a fresh, spiritual, more optimistic perspective. She wasn't afraid of my "dark nights of the soul." She saw the good in me through all of it. What a gift.

She also introduced me to German New Medicine, which views Lyme disease completely differently than any current paradigm. This has freed me immensely and helped me quit holding on so tight in fear, so much that for the first time in three years, I said "yes!" to my daughters when they asked if

they could go to the Outdoor Education Center this past fall!
I followed through and let them go, even though so much
within me (my amygdala especially!) was saying, "No!
Don't do it! It's not safe!" (Reminder: Don't believe
everything you think.)

I did some Emotional Freedom Technique (EFT) tapping
that I learned from Amy Scher's group phone calls. That
helped lots.

Saying "yes!" to my daughters was a major turning point for
me. It was empowering and exhilarating, going through the
fear… and coming out on the other side, triumphant, having
done something I thought was impossible! It got even better
upon hearing how excited my daughters were when they
came back from a day in the forest, beaming and bursting at
the seams to tell me about what they learned and saw. It
brought me to tears. For a long time, I didn't think I'd ever
let my kids go back into the woods again.

I still haven't gone back into the woods, but I believe now
that it won't take heaven for me to do that.

If there's one piece of advice that I'd give, above all, it
would be to follow a path of love, to avoid, as often as
possible, things that incite fear, hate, or victimizing. Let go
of your need to have certain outcomes in certain timeframes.
Instead, I would encourage you to open your heart, follow
your intuition.

Never stop questioning. Don't simply follow the herd

mindlessly.

The way practitioners and others treat you is important. Surround yourself as often as possible with positive energy.

Don't be afraid of your own darkness. It is temporary and passing, like clouds in the big, beautiful sky.

What if we fired our inner critic and hired a cheerleader instead? What if we strove for self-love?

Healing is always possible and it's much more than simply the absence of physical symptoms. Never give up. Keep on.

While Lyme is a part of my journey, a part of my life story, it is simply that. I honor it. I thank it. But... it does not define me. My being open to it and listening to it has helped shape me and grow me. It has revealed truths and opened doorways to healing and transformation, but it does not define me. I am so much more than just "Lyme." And so, I humbly and gladly drop the label, and any others, to make more space, more room for the real me to continue to emerge.

I'm Lisa.
I'm not Lisa the Lutheran.
I'm not Lisa with Lyme.
I'm not a "Lymie."
I'm not a victim, nor a martyr.
No labels, no boxes necessary.
I'm just Lisa.
And that is

Way more than
ENOUGH.

Lisa is a Midwest girl born and raised in Wisconsin. She has two brothers and two sisters (one who is her twin), all born in just three and a half years! She went to college & ended up with degrees in psychology and education/teaching. She also met and married her very funny husband during that time, and now they have three children (ages five, eight, & 12).

She is currently a stay-at-home mom. She has an insatiable curiosity and continues to read and learn lots every day. Her passions/interests are many and include: math, the brain, children, families, education, relationships, holistic/integrative healing, spirituality, mindfulness, and Nonviolent Communication/peace-making.

She also loves to laugh, be silly, sing, dance, read, and enjoy the beauty & is-ness of nature/wildlife.

Michelle

I first realized that something was off with my health in 1988, during college. I could not stay awake in the afternoon and was completely exhausted. Health issues manifested and changed over the years. According to the doctors, there was nothing wrong. I knew that some day I would have to figure it out. Changing symptoms by the minute, day, week, month or year, I knew was not normal.

I was an athlete on the Canadian National Development Freestyle ski team for moguls in the early 90's and had many injuries. I always thought that the pains, joint aches and muscular tension that pulled my body out of alignment were related to my injuries. I also could not perform under competition or exam pressure. I almost always crashed within the first five moguls in a competition, as my legs would not bend properly. In training, I would never crash. I learned that the bacteria of Lyme was an opportunist, took advantage of any form of stress and migrated into old injuries or weaknesses in the body and affected the nervous system.

During my fifth season of working as a hiking guide, I felt zapped of all my energy. I was too tired to do my usual climbing or biking after work or on days off. A few months later, I deteriorated quickly and I thought I was going to die. Six months later, someone suggested that I probably had Lyme disease. Most people turn a blind eye to Lyme and I was fortunate enough to be diagnosed by someone that also had it. Thank goodness for other sufferers who are educating the general public and the medical community.

I went from working and exercising everyday to doing less and less over the years. I always tried to fix whatever the issue was. Lots of physiotherapy, chiropractic, ART (Active Release Technique), massage, rolfing, IMS (Intra-Muscular Stimulation), acupuncture, cranial sacral and tons of stretching which eventually turned to yoga. Symptoms migrated from one area to another and my quest to understand my body always kept me puzzled and busy.

After being on antibiotics for four out of the last five years during treatment for Lyme, Bartonella and Babesia, I am mostly feeling like a normal human being these days.

One of the greatest lessons I've learned is self-discipline and focus. I have been motivated to keep my body in good running order. Going gluten free, dairy free, eating clean and avoiding sugar was a major key to getting better. I put in the time to rehabilitate my body to get the physical tension under control by rolling on foam rollers and different size balls. This was crucial for me to function properly as the muscle tension constantly pulled everything out of alignment and created other issues. I believe that Lyme disease has helped me have excellent body awareness (except when nerve damage stopped some muscles from working properly) and excel in sports.

I can't say enough about yoga and meditation as it has helped both physically and mentally. Proper breathing is the key to a healthy life and getting through the pain. Thinking of the breath and taking full inhales and exhales throughout the day gave me a good idea where my body holds tension. I would breathe into the area to release the chronic tightness. Yoga is a lifestyle that can be adopted anywhere. Focusing on the breath, in the moment with no thoughts, as the body moves and flows, is a healing practice. Try what I call household yoga. Bring awareness to the breath and movements in your body during everyday activities. Always be mindful of your posture. Good body alignment is a key factor to reduce pain and alleviate stress on organs, joints, muscles, tendons, ligaments and nervous system.

You can be creative and incorporate stretches into everyday living. For example, try to do lunges the next time you vacuum, tree pose the next time you do the dishes or a forward bend when you go to pick something off the floor. Possibilities are endless. I find myself creating new ways to stretch, depending on what my body needs.

It's important to keep the lymph nodes moving. Without detoxing, there is no treatment success. Lyme gives you thick blood, which makes activity even more important. When I exercised, the first half hour would make me feel horrible, but then I would start to feel better. Stick with it. Things will improve and you will get stronger. Acupuncture also benefits by helping to keep the energy moving through the organs and meridians.

The most difficult part of this illness is the lack of diagnoses and treatment in the medical community. This lack of awareness and education becomes isolating and sadly leaves one socially deprived. Education is slowly happening that will someday bring more understanding and less stress to the sufferers. I got through this difficult time by the healing and loving purr of my cat, Bugaboo. Animals seem to know what's going on.

I have always been a spiritual person, studying Buddhism and yoga. Over the years I felt as if something was eating my spirit. This, in the end, made me spiritually stronger than ever. I suggest to everyone to find and read a spiritual book (such as Light on Life by B.K.S. Iyengar and Seeking the Heart of Wisdom by Joseph Goldstein and Jack Kornfield), especially when you feel like you are losing your life. I also realized the importance of having faith that you will get your life back. Giving up is not an option.

If treatment is not working like it should or reaches a plateau, try adding a supplement or change your diet. I spent numerous hours a day researching things that could improve my health. I highly recommend reading Dr. Horowitz's book "Why Can't I Get Better." This would have saved me months of research. He gives the chronic illness sufferer 16 different avenues that can be addressed to get back to optimal health.

I credit Lyme disease for making me tough and strong, even though I lost a lot of strength during the peak of my illness. I would be in "go mode" when most people would be sitting on the couch. This led to an internal strength. My mental headspace kept me moving and exercising. It is key to be positive.

A good tip for anyone starting out is to not expect the doctors to fix you. You have to put the time in and do it yourself. It can be a full time job. You ultimately are responsible for your own healing.

The most difficult part of Lyme disease is it robs you of everything you used to be able to do. Going from a high performance athlete to barely moving off the couch was not something I was proud of. The greatest lesson I learned here is to live in the moment and accept where you are right now. This is where happiness is found. Forget about the past. Forget about what you used to do, friends or family that were not there for you or anything that takes you to the past. Forget about what your future might look like. Live in the now, do things to improve your quality of life, stick to it, and have faith that things will improve. Have patience and you will get your life back!

Michelle is a mountain girl that lives in the Canadian Rockies. She loves to climb, bike, ski, hike, do yoga, live life by the moment, and teach all that she has learned. "I believe I contracted Lyme through birth and started trying to figure out what was wrong with me twenty seven years ago. I do my best to educate others about Lyme disease and have hope that the mainstream medical community will turn the corner and start to diagnose and treat it."

Melinda Lippert

In June of 2008, I had an intensely angry bite that refused to heal at the base of my skull, followed by strange symptoms with no obvious cause. They grew in number, frequency, and severity.

Standard Western medicine could not diagnose or fix me. I had classic textbook Lyme disease, but I wasn't lucky enough to have the narrowly defined magic combination of bands on the standard Western Blot. My life was utterly derailed by chronic Lyme and co-infections that raged misdiagnosed for over 3 years.

Countless doctor visits and several Western Blots later, my doctor said the test result was negative – again – and the only explanation for my long list of bizarre symptoms was the fact that I was a stressed-out perfectionistic mother of two kids. She suggested I start drinking wine or take anti-depressants. I wanted to slug her for the insulting judgment, but the lymph nodes in my armpits were so swollen and sore I couldn't swing my arm. And my balance was so wobbly I would have fallen off the exam table.

Instead I listened to my intuition, which was screaming because I'd ignored it so long. I asked to see the lab report for myself. It had two positive bands, but the wrong combination. I demanded a copy of every lab report for the past three years and I kissed that doctor's condescending ass goodbye forever.

I often wish I'd known to question medical authority and ask to see my test results at the onset. I'd be telling a very different story. But we all learn our lessons in our own time. I would never have evolved without walking the path of chronic Lyme. The many lessons I learned taught me self-advocacy, faith, compassion, wisdom, strength, and ignited the light of my inner healer. I now wish that you may benefit from my experiences as you navigate your own healing journey.

My lessons were many.

I learned to stop relying on doctors to fix me.
If I wanted to be well again, I had to take charge of my own healing. I read every book available on healing Lyme disease, (not politics or personal accounts of suffering, but healing). I put into practice what resonated with me and worked for me. I disregarded what didn't resonate or didn't help. I learned to trust that I know myself and my body better than any doctor ever could.

I found integrative health care practitioners who understood Lyme disease.
Yes, it was expensive. No, insurance did not cover it. I chose practitioners carefully, listening to my intuition. The prestigious super-expensive LLMD known for IV antibiotic cocktails wasn't right for me. I combined many different alternative therapies with good results.

Proper diagnosis is just the beginning.
Healing Lyme is not a straightforward path and is much

more than killing spirochetes. I learned to piece together a complex puzzle of pathogen reduction, nutrition, detox strategies, immune and hormone regulation, and emotional healing. I spent a fortune on things that didn't work and occasionally found things that did work. My healing was often three steps forward and two steps back.

Endless worry over ominous numbers decreases your immune function.

Diagnostic tests are helpful, but don't base your life on your latest CD-57 count. You don't need every test, supplement, protocol, medical device, healing tool, or the trendiest doctor in order to heal. We are all different. What works for someone else or all the doctor's other patients may or may not work for you. Trust in your ability to make good decisions about what you need.

Clinging tightly to symptoms is not the path to wellness.

Your focus determines your reality. When people learn I had Lyme disease, they respond in one of two ways:

1. Really? I have Lyme, too! Tell me your Lyme history. What were your symptoms? Were they like my symptoms? Right now I've got…

2. Really? I have Lyme, too. Tell me – what did you do to get well?

Their response is an accurate indicator of where they are in their healing journey. I won't dredge up the old symptom list. It's in my past and I'm not looking in that direction. I'd rather discuss how to get well. Focus your every intention on healing and your path will unfold.

When symptoms are severe, stop fighting.
Surrender. Rest. Then shift your focus away from your symptoms. Listen to soothing music or watch comedies. I liked to play cards with my kids and listen to their stories. Those quiet moments were true blessings from Lyme. The stillness helped me find balance. Now that I'm well, I make time to connect and recharge.

It's healing for your spirit to occasionally allow yourself to eat the cookie or beautiful homemade bread.
Savor every bite despite the gluten. Return to your special diet tomorrow.

Gratitude always gets you more of the good stuff.
Appreciate all you have. Notice every improvement.

Yes, you need emotional healing, even if you think you don't.
Chronic illness has many underlying emotional ties and you won't heal until you address them. You will heal much faster if you address them in the beginning rather than later. I could have prevented years of suffering if I'd accepted this concept before my fifth year of Lyme.

Stress, fear, and worry are the biggest hazards to my health. They're even worse than microbes. Four years into this disease, I'd made some great healing progress. Life threw a curve ball that gave me concrete proof how emotions impact health. My husband's job was eliminated. Worry and fear ruled my life. My health spiraled backward. God sends us lessons so we learn what we most need to know. I'd learned a lot about physical health, but at the same time ignored the emotional component. I needed this fundamental lesson to understand the detrimental impact of stress and fear and the importance of emotional and spiritual healing.

Most Lyme books have sections devoted to underlying emotional ties to illness and how healing old emotional patterns is crucial for achieving wellness. I skipped those chapters because I thought it didn't apply to me. That was written for other chronic Lyme people, I thought. I finally recognized that stress was my physical undoing and saw how that had been true my entire life. From early childhood, I'd internalized every hurt. Whenever I felt tremendous stress, my body responded with physical illness. It was a well-rehearsed subconscious pattern. Plus, I worried like a champ. I carried my own worries and also took on the worries of those I loved. I often made myself sick with worry – literally! It was obvious in hindsight.

I'd like to say I accepted the insight with grace, but no, I beat myself up even more for the ways in which I'd unknowingly contributed to illness, the ways in which illness had served me. At times, illness had been a convenient excuse to avoid facing or doing difficult things. Then came an epiphany. I had in my hand what I now consider the most vital piece of my healing puzzle: if my mind-body connection was so powerful it created these problems, my mind-body connection was powerful enough to resolve them! I had the ability to actually do something about it!

I worked to correct the underlying emotional components of unhealed traumas and limiting beliefs. Traditional talk therapy and rehashing the same stories only reinforced the issues and made me feel worse. My answer came from the emerging field of energy psychology. With Emotional Freedom Technique (EFT), the Emotion Code, and a few other techniques, I uncovered and addressed the issues, one by one. It was deep and at times painful to face, but far better to acknowledge it in order to release and heal, than to continue to deny it and stuff it down. I still experience worry, fear, and stress, but now I acknowledge and release instead of internalizing.

True healing encompasses physical, emotional, and spiritual components.
Addressing these aspects together was the final key to regulating my immune and digestive systems. Most of my emotional traumas and energetic blocks were centered in my digestive organs. Much of my hormonal function normalized by removing emotional energies and disturbances located in and around my glands.

For five years, all I wanted every moment was to once again be comfortable in my own body: to move without pain, eat without sickness or allergies, sleep peacefully, think clearly, write and speak articulately, run errands without getting lost or exhausting myself, to have a social life, and to care for the emotional and physical needs of my family. In the darkest moments I felt misunderstood, lost, isolated, and drained:

physically, spiritually, emotionally, and financially. I'd lost my former self. But it was there in the darkness that I found the wisdom, faith, healing, and inner strength that created the spark from which a different and better life grew.

It's difficult to say that Lyme disease was a gift, but I definitely see how illness was a necessary step, a life lesson that led me to where God and The Universe ultimately intended. I discovered what it took to heal myself at the core, and I went through professional trainings to deepen my healing skills. I came to see energetic emotional healing as my calling in life and I now use my first-hand knowledge to help others heal.

Lyme is behind me. I'm in the final phases of healing the residual damage. It takes time and it happens one layer at a time. I'm at 98% and I know 100% is absolutely within reach. If I ever face another serious illness, I will stop and ask what imbalance allowed it to manifest, what is my body trying to tell me? I trust in my ability to heal, for the ultimate healing comes from within. This is true for you as well. Have faith.

Melinda Lippert specializes in emotional healing and the mind-body connection. She believes that we all have deep within us an infinite capacity to heal and we are all meant to lead lives filled with joy. She is a certified Emotion Code practitioner, EFT (Tapping) practitioner, yoga teacher (200 hour CYT), an ordained minister of holistic healing, and has a Bachelor's degree in biology. She works with clients to heal and release negative emotions, neutralize past traumas,

*and break ties to chronic illness while accessing and
balancing the body's energetic meridian system. These
negative energies often contribute to emotional and physical
symptoms. Releasing and neutralizing them allows the body
to achieve a state of balance where health, happiness, and
wellness flourish. She lives near Albany, NY with her
husband, their son and daughter, and two cats.
www.melindalippert.com*

Julia Shay Tuchman

Adam and I are standing outside a Chinese restaurant at night, waiting for a bus. The distinctive smell of Szechwan cuisine escaping from the restaurant onto the street surrounds me. It fills my nose and sends a signal to my brain that I am hungry. I start to cry. I am standing on Second Avenue crying because I can't eat. Adam sees me crying and without a word he holds my hand. The smell of the food is so strong and exquisite that he need not question why I am crying. He knows. This was seven years ago. It had only been a year since I once again lost the ability to swallow solid foods again.

I once stared at a woman briskly walking down the street— her yoga bag hanging from her back as she ate an apple. She looked at me most likely wondering why I was staring. I stared because to walk and eat at the same time is a wonder to me, as if I just saw the most amazing magic act right in front of me. I see her take a bite and then another and the apple slowly disappears. I wonder if she knows how miraculous it all is, but I am sure she does not. I know when I could eat I did not know how miraculous it was either.

I watch in awe at a man cycling down First Avenue on his bike while eating a slice of pizza.
"Wow!" I say aloud. Biking and eating all at the same time seems incredible, and yet he does it with ease. I watch kids as they eat cupcakes while they walk or gobble up bagels as they play. I see how they can even skip while eating as if it is the most natural thing in the world. I guess it is. These are

things I never noticed when I could eat.

In Manhattan there is a restaurant on every block, often more than one. The smells of cuisine from all over the world linger outside of the incredible number of restaurants in the borough: Indian, Italian, Chinese, Israeli, Burmese, Thai, Soul food. Often all the aromas join together as if in a dance. Each smell pokes me in the gut and my heart. "Here, look what you can't have, Julia" they say to me. "Look what is not for you!"

Food is everywhere. Often, when I smell the heavenly aromas coming out of restaurants I hear my stomach talking to me, not understanding. If my mouth is salivating, why then do I not go into the restaurant and get that piece of pizza? I can't. I can't swallow it. "Go in there and order that piece of white pizza with onions," says my stomach that for some reason sounds like a grumpy old man. "That guy in there is eating a slice? What's wrong with you, kid?" How do I explain this to my stomach? I can hardly understand all this myself. "I know you want that piece of pizza with all of your heart or gut" I silently reply. "But, the transit to get it to you is faulty right now. There is glitch in the system." All I hear back is my stomach making hungry gurgling sounds. The smell of pizza does that to my stomach.

There is shock and many times I have to say to myself, "Okay Julia, This is what happened: this virus or mold infection damaged your nerves or brain, and then you lost your ability to swallow solid food." I had dealt with CFS and MCS for so many years, and then this loss again seemed too much for me. I go to NYU Langone Hospital to get another barium swallow test. The nurse and doctor watch from the x-ray room and I can see their faces through the glass partition as I swallow concoctions of chalky barium. The nurse who reminded me of a blonde Betty Boop character is trying to be funny "I've seen worse," she says.

A week later my neurologist enters her office with the test results in her hands. The look on her face is one of helplessness and no answers. "You have a big problem," she says. That was it. There was no "You have a problem Ms. Tuchman and this is how we are going to fix it: two hours in the operating room and then pizza!" Cheers and applause. Joyous cinematic music used for the life-changing scene begins to play in the background. This would be fixed in no time. No, None of that. They have no cure and no answers.

While walking down a Manhattan street, I stop at the window of a cozy looking Chinese restaurant. I watch a family eating at a large table laughing smiling and I am brought back in my mind to my childhood when my parents would bring my siblings and I to Tung Sing. We would eat the wonderful food while the staff would often have fights in the kitchen—throwing plates of food and arguing in Chinese. It was all wonderful and magical, but far more than I even knew then. I did not know about such things as not being able to swallow food then nor illness. I knew Tung Sing was that place where egg rolls, spare ribs and those crunchy friend noodles were always waiting for me. I watched this family now through the window - my mind taking me back to that restaurant so many years ago and the feeling of family, laughter and food. I wanted that again. I snapped out of the memory of ghosts of Chinese meals past and continued walking on.

I felt left out—an outsider from this important part of life, this physical need, this social need—and worst of all, this might be for life. "But you are alive," my father will often remind me. "Where there is life there is hope," he says to me often. "It came back once before," he says "It can come back again." He is right. Mila, the holocaust survivor who lives at his assisted living facility holds my hand when I first meet her and tells me, "If your eyes are still open there is hope." I listen to her. She would know.

There are silent screams that fill me when the deprivation feels too much. I walk by a restaurant on one of those days. I am on the other side of the windowpane separating me from the diners, and I pass by one table after another filled with people eating lunch. A woman about my age eats a grilled cheese sandwich, a favorite of mine as a kid. I used to put French fries in the sandwich with ketchup. People would laugh at my odd combination, but I loved it. I am brought back to my childhood and to my days when eating was effortless and life seemed sweeter. I begin to cry. I instinctively put my hand up to my throat in a loving gentle swoop and say aloud, "I love you Julia." My voice sounds kind like a mother comforting her child. With each table I pass I say, "I love you, Julia. I love you." Another table with a family eating, "I love you. Julia". Tears fall as this kindness engulfs me. I was starving for this loving kindness to myself as much as I was hungry for food. This was not a planned "I love you Julia" after reading a self-help book or even a conscious decision. It was not what I was supposed to do or what I was told to do. It came from the depths of my soul. It spoke to my heart, then to my voice box and brain as well, and out of my mouth with no conscious thought. An "I love you" escaped from me into the Manhattan air and then back to my own ears. I was filling myself up. I was nourishing myself.

I had lost so much, but I had this gentle touch to my throat and the kind words to myself in spite of it all. There was power in that. There is something about invisible disability that is doubly hurtful. Nobody sees it, or understands it, and so they judge. We then in turn judge ourselves. I have judged myself too and I have beaten myself up over and over as if I were somehow responsible for all the years of illness and seemingly endless knock-downs. But on that day, when I passed those people eating and touched my throat, I was speaking kind and loving words to myself and that choice was the healing. There is power in that choice.

Last week I arrived early for a doctor's appointment, and I sat with my eyes closed in the waiting room to rest. The secretaries were talking for a half hour about which restaurant they wanted to go to for a large family get-together. They mentioned every type of food and every type of restaurant available in New York. One was eating McDonald's and another was eating a sandwich as they discussed their plans. I had my thermos of protein shake. I was surprised at how neutral I felt. I was hearing them talk, but not attached to what they said. I let the words flow over me and through me.

"You really want to test me, God," I said aloud to the ceiling of the empty waiting room as they continued talking about my favorite meals. I was assuming God was in the ceiling of a doctor's office. I am certain the ceiling of waiting rooms hear many prayers.

I touched my throat and sent myself love again. I also sent blessings to my liquefied food and went to a place of gratitude for it. It was getting easier. I even gave myself acknowledgement for how far I have come through all of this. There is a grace, I have found in these sacred moments of self–love and acceptance, which even this illness can never take away.

"I love you Julia." I say as I touch my throat. I love you even if you can't eat normally. I love you even if this is forever. I love you even if this all heals tomorrow. I even love you if this never heals. I touch my throat and send it love. That I can do. I can do that.

Julia Shay Tuchman is a writer living in NYC. After a bout of mononucleosis, she was diagnosed with CFS/MCS and experienced nerve damage from a virus affecting the ability to swallow solid food. Julia writes about her experiences and of the lessons in self-love no matter what our circumstance. www.JuliaTuchman.com

Michelle Sinclair

In October 2013, I found myself in Darkness. I had spent the last three solid years chasing, identifying, attacking and constantly adjusting and readjusting my everything to Lyme and associated vector-borne infections. The weight and breadth of the Darkness was all-encompassing; my body was broken, my mind mush, my spirit crushed, my future unsure, my bank account negative and my support system exhausted.

Over the years, I have found that my Lyme journey is so similar to so many I have seen and heard. I had some odd, though not debilitating, certainly curious and unrelated symptomology throughout childhood and my young adult life. Nothing showed in routine tests and for a young, healthy person I was dismissed. I also dismissed these things even as they added up because my family physician and other specialists were not picking anything up. I had a series of symptoms in college while I was not insured and just dealt with them, figuring it was the stress of my schedule. After a somewhat difficult first pregnancy and the traumatic delivery of my daughter, things started to really go downhill. After the birth, we suffered a few tragic personal losses, traumas and victimizations. At a six-month baby wellness checkup, after refusing four times in the same visit, I was 'convinced' by her pediatrician to get my first (and only) flu shot. It turned into a non-stop three years of confusing, scary and debilitating symptoms and the total breakdown of my body and mind due to massive infection. Of course, during this time I was insured. Regardless, we had spent nearly $150,000 out-of-pocket diagnosing and toying with this blasted set of infections in just over three years. Over 70 doctors and specialists saw me before I was clinically diagnosed (followed up by tests for Lyme and multiple co-infections). To many of these medical 'professionals' it was clear that all I had was "Depression, Not Otherwise Specified", "Fibromyalgia", "Chronic Fatigue Syndrome" and "Myofascial Pain Syndrome." I had more than one family member accuse me of misleading family and doctors while merely seeking prescriptions. The two problems with these diagnoses and judgments were, 1) I knew in my being-- in that place where I really am who I am, that that was utter bullshit, and 2) in March of 2013, I was finally validated medically via blood test in addition to my prior clinical diagnosis that I was in fact positive for Lyme and many, many co-infections.

It is an easy place to get to the Darkness. What I was totally naive about, however, was how easily it is for the Darkness to utterly descend without realizing it. When I noticed it, it was the Darkness of a cavern one visits on vacation to a special cave system, where fish are devoid of pigment and blind and the creatures below must adapt in total lack of Light. My eyes must have adapted to the slow settling of Darkness as it blanketed me.

I mean, I knew it sucked to be so sick for so long that I wasn't sure some days if I would wake up the next morning. Even when I wasn't sure my husband was a believer, I had found online support groups which helped with the insomnia and the constant search for what pathogen to target next by other's advice. I had friends that not only believed me, but had real experience with all of this mess I was in. These friends knew so much and were so into this world that they traded symptom posters as though the Bartonella poster with the typo and one-off color mistake would make tens of thousands someday on Antique Roadshow. This wasn't Darkness, this was sick people doing all they could to educate the Freshman Lyme Class into this new reality. I love these people. I AM these people.

Looking back, I realized that I never really read one thing that really explained that someone had been successfully treated--ever--from Lyme and co-infections. I have recently heard that the reason those improving are so silent, when they improve, is that first, they are now away from the computer more often and living again presumably. Also, second, having lived this hell, they fear that the sharing of their success could have an enormously negative effect on those in the midst of the darkness and rather than inspire, send them further into Darkness and depression. I know that I, myself, have thought about it this way as well.

After all that time, money and stress I decided that I could no longer be Lyme's bitch. I decided to maintain my illness out of a doctor's office at home, for whatever time I had left. I was being pragmatic. I was broke and exhausted and deflated and ready to spend quality time with my family out of a car traveling to a specialist's office. I continued the grief counseling I had started months earlier. I started to read again. I decided I was going to be patient both with me and my illness. I realized that things may have to be re-read (ten times), glasses and plates will be dropped, I will trip, and I may not get out of the house even once per month. I was okay with all of this. I accepted it. I had the little person that had only ever known me ill telling me to drink my ozone, take my nap, and use my heating pad. The husband I about divorced, due to the rage, let me just rest and he took care of everything (I am not sure how, but he did an amazing job. I love you, Grant.) With their permission and my decision, I let my whole self truly rest for the first time in a long time.

It came suddenly. In that tourist trap you visit with the family over fourth grade summer, the guide instructs you all to turn out your lights. The total and absolute Darkness of that great room in the belly of the earth astounds you and sucks the breath right out of your lungs. The guide strikes a single matchstick. A tiny speck of light illuminates the cavernous absence of all light. The Darkness must retreat, even from the tiniest Light. In that sulfur-smoke moment, there was Light, yes, but there was also perspective and depth and meaning and love and an understanding. And there was pain. It was hard to actually feel all the pain. I was suddenly able to see it, work with it, dismantle it and sort it. It. Was. Amazing. As suddenly as the Light interrupted The Dark, I realized I wasn't merely fighting Lyme and co-infections, but I was involved in a epic battle of will. When no one or almost no one believes what you have no reason to mislead them about, The Light is that much more evident and immense when it finally pierces through. A match in a cave can feel so comforting and warm compared to that vast breath-sucking Dark. That one match light that I was given is what motivated me to seek out the tiniest matches of hope to compound and grow this Light within the

Darkness and to recognize all the tiny matches of hope and motivation strewn all about me.

No, I am not 100%-before-I-got-sick-well, and I know I may never be. But, that is okay now; I am at peace with that possibility. I also have peace from knowing that there is always hope. Within the last three or four months, I have witnessed many of my dearest Lymies, all of whom were bed-bound and disabled, start to heal! Quietly we would sheepishly answer each other's texts, "I don't want to jinx this, but I am actually doing really well! Seeing such improvement!" We are hiking, growing our businesses, cooking for our families and participating in the greater community again--it is glorious.

Just like the stigma with mental health in general, there is serious stigma around sharing the success stories, even the small victories, with others that are in the trenches of The Darkness. Can we change this? Can those experiencing these improvements start to band together, provide an inspirational support for others without fear? I think we can. I think if we take the time to offer encouragement, show these Freshman how some of the undergraduates have changed, it might take that stigma and desperation away from the infected brain. I think it could be a great comfort if more of those of us showing some improvements shouted this to everyone, "THERE IS HOPE! DO NOT GIVE UP! IT GETS BETTER!!" Enough of us need to proclaim this in a universal, loving and encouraging tone.
If there is one thing I know about Lymies and the chronically ill, it is their immense compassion and empathy for

suffering. It is time for the Lyme community to support each other by sharing, with all of these souls and bodies others stuck in The Darkness, that while we do know all about The Dark, but we can also tell you a little about The Light.

I would offer this in summary: Through this process of illness, misdiagnosis, disbelief, mistreatment, treatment, and healing, I would say to anyone going through this either as a patient, caretaker or onlooker that it gets better. It gets much better. You can live again and flourish. You can be both chronically ill simultaneously with being as happy or at peace as you have ever been. I know you can because I am. While you are in the midst of Darkness, remember that it gets better. If the rage or depression gets too heavy, reach out to this community of amazing, sympathetic and caring people. We are out there and we will remind you we get better.

Michelle Sinclair is a freelance illustrator, photographer, designer and native Arizonan. A Lyme advocate and "Chronic Lymie," she is passionate about spreading the awareness of and assistance for chronic auto-immune-disordered patients everywhere.
http://www.etsy.com/shop/MichStudios

Gail Lynn Heil

July of 2013, I left my home in New York to visit relatives in New Jersey. A warm sunny week ahead delighted me as I was embarking on a road trip with my daddy and step mom. I was having a happy, healthy, vibrant, and carefree time until four days later when I awoke early that morning feeling a little "off", with some pressure in my chest that took my breath away. I also started experiencing headaches, body aches, exhaustion, and tingling sensations in my head. As a Reiki practitioner, I began self-healing until the symptoms subsided, but they would only return later. I was normally very healthy and didn't know what was wrong, but did know that I was coming down with something. The pain then became so unbearable that it wasn't long before we decided we should head home. Never had it occurred to me that this was the beginning of a life-changing event.

The next day, after a short urgent care visit, the doctor diagnosed me with plantar fasciitis. He prescribed Naproxen Sodium and urged me to get some "supportive" shoes. I began the prescription, but the flu-like symptoms continued. The next week, my ankles looked the size of an elephants so I went to see my doctor and was given a prescription for Tramadol, an order for blood work to be done, and a new "diagnosis" of gout. Days passed and I gained new symptoms. I was scared, wondering what was happening to me, and decided to visit the Healing Temple for spiritual healing. I sat with tears rolling down my face, asking God to heal my body.

The following week was a nightmare with new and worsening symptoms. I was taken to the Emergency Room and admitted to the hospital where I was hooked up to an EKG and IV, had more blood drawn, was given a dose of prednisone and offered Hydrocodone for pain. By evening, the doctor sent me home with medication, after telling me that my blood test results were fine and to call back in a week for test results of the West Nile, EEE, and a Western Blot. I could not believe what I was hearing! They were letting me go without knowing what was wrong! I could barely walk! How they could dismiss me so easily? I wanted answers! I staggered out of our local ER, crying out in pain, frustration, and fear.

Once home, I began a frantic research of all my symptoms, the medical terminology of the blood work results, and possible causes of what was happening to my body. I began learning about SED rates, CBC, ANA, and every acronym that was placed on any medical record that I was now accumulating. I was determined to find my own diagnosis and healing treatment. I prayed hourly, crying out to God, wanting to understand what lessons I needed to see in all this. I talked with teachers and friends whom were expert healers and mediums, looking for answers and insight, taking suggestions, trying various recommended healing modalities, and receiving prayers of healing. Nothing was going to stop me from finding a solution, a diagnosis, a healing modality, something to help me see "the lesson", and make me well again.

Medically, I was displeased with the various diagnoses and

prescriptions thrown at me, so I began looking for more natural courses, with my alternative health practitioners, who recommended herbs and various methods to boost my immune system. I was told that bacteria, from Lyme disease, had invaded my body, along with two other co-infections, and if I followed the recommendations from my spirit doctors, which included Amoxicillin, I would begin to heal.

At the same time, my family doctor referred me to a Rheumatologist and I immediately knew this was NOT the place for me, as I had neither arthritis nor Lupus, which the Rheumatologist suggested. After this, I decided to stop taking the prednisone, that my family doctor kept pushing, and all pain pills. My healing routine now consisted of a combination of diet, exercise, spiritual practice, and the Amoxicillin.

My next referral was to Cleveland Clinic. After a few hours of questioning and seventeen vials of blood, they finished up and left me with a departing statement of, "You can check online for your test results". After two weeks of frantically trying to decipher test results online, I finally called and spoke with the specialist I saw who merely said, "Whatever you are doing, keep it up because all your tests are improving, so whatever it is you are doing is helping." "That's it?!" I thought as I hung up the phone. "That's all they have to offer me?"

Six weeks of pain, fear, confusion, and fighting not only for my physical body, but my sanity as well, all came crashing down on me. I'd hit a brick wall and I was determined more than ever to take charge of my own health. I went to the Healing Temple, changed my diet to raw foods and began a mission of healing mind, body, and soul. I prayed, meditated, and spent time alone with God. Day by day, I fought to heal. I felt alone fighting this, yet friends and family online gave me strength. I spent hours on Facebook reading inspirational readings and posts. I asked for prayers. I read every article I could put my hands on. I was gaining strength, but after my two weeks of Amoxicillin was up, my symptoms returned.

The antibiotics helped, as shown by the herxheimer reactions, but every time I started to make gains, the Amoxicillin ran out and I was brought back down. When I finally broke down and called my family doctor, I explained how the Amoxicillin helped, feeling I had to convince him my symptoms were real. I told him about my naturopath's thoughts of Lyme disease, and he only laughed, stating that I tested negative on Lyme. He then proceeded to tell me that he would prescribe the Amoxicillin for me to try one more time, but when it didn't work, I would try his route of prednisone for the inflammation and an anti-depressant for my "stress." I was flabbergasted by what sounded like a deal he was trying to make, but knew I needed it, so I accepted his "deal." I began my third round of Amoxicillin for another two weeks.

While insomnia gave me time to diligently research, I discovered an online documentary, "Under Our Skin." Within minutes, I was sobbing. The stories I heard and witnessed were *my* story (why was this happening, feeling like I was going to die, it's all in your head, knowing something is attacking your body but no physician could help, relentless pain, etc.). I had finally found answers. I don't know why it made me happy, but knowing someone out there could relate, that I wasn't crazy, and that this was real, was a relief.

I awoke the next morning asking the question "why?" and heard, "because you are being led to grow spiritually." It finally dawned on me that all this time I kept looking for answers outside of myself. I ran like a beggar to so many, while I should have looked within, I knew where the answers were, but I didn't practice what I knew. The body and higher-self know what to do to heal and how to lead the way; I just needed to listen. I was not valuing my own self, my own inner light and consciousness.

Then one day, I was given the name of a Lyme Literate doctor. The moment I looked into his eyes, I knew that he was *not* a doctor but a healer who was put onto my path to help me the rest of the way on my healing journey. After two visits, blood work and MRI results, he gave me the diagnosis of Lyme disease. All I could respond with is, "Yes doc, I know. I've seen it, I've felt it, and I was told months back by my 'helpers', but I let fear and pain own me." Time to take back my life.

I began a new prescription of Doxycycline and through trial and error, eastern and western medicine, and days of fear and pain, I have made it!

Perseverance, prayer, spiritual healing, Reiki, energy work, change of diet, natural supplements, staying positive, meditation, affirmations, love of those around me and my LLMD, Any given day I feel weak, I scan the pages of Louise Hay and after reading one affirmation after another, my soul is strengthened. One favorite I've taken from her and other inspirational teachers and meshed together is, "I am the author and creator of my life story." When I don't like how it is going...I yell out, "PLOT TWIST!!"

The most beneficial change in my diet came from the words of Hippocrates, "Let food be thy medicine and medicine be thy food." I believe my body can heal itself given proper nutrition. If it's not good for my body, then I've cut it out. Eating sugars, dairy, processed foods, canned foods and carbs is like feeding fish (the bacteria from Lyme disease being the fish). I drink green smoothies every morning with raw food as much as I can. When I cheat and have chocolate, I unfortunately, pay for it with more symptoms such as headaches, body aches or fogginess. Nutrition makes such a great difference.

On those days when it's really hard, I ask for prayers from family and friends. I believe in the power of prayer. I do self-Reiki, meditate, listen to music that uplifts me, call a friend who lifts me. I do whatever it takes. Some days, a good cry is needed, and then I get back up and fight. I remind myself there are people who have it worse than I and I kick myself for being a victim.

Lastly, I listen to my higher consciousness, by just sitting in the quiet and listening. When I want to know what to do, I sit and ask my higher conscious, my higher self, and an answer will come. I just simply need to ask the right question and then listen! And then take action!

I am on my way back! I am grateful to so many who have guided me, prayed for me, supported me, and simply loved me through it all. I am blessed. One of life's greatest lessons I learned was to listen to my own inner guidance. And, to never give up! I offer a prayer, to all those who have suffered through Lyme and the co-infections or any chronic illness... keep up the fight! Go within and listen to your higher consciousness; just sit in the quiet and listen! When you want to know what to do, sit and ask your higher conscious, your self, and an answer will come. We just simply need to ask the right question and then listen! And then take action! Anything you truly desire is possible!

Gail Lynn Heil has her MS in Elementary Education. She devotes her summers to serving the Lily Dale Community as a workshop coordinator and as a Spiritual Healer in The Healing Temple. She is an Ordained Minister, a Reiki Practitioner, Spiritual Counselor, Medium, and a member of the Lily Dale Assembly. She will be leading a workshop in Lily Dale August 2014 called, "Take Back Your Life."

Jenny Rush

"Passing through the eye of the needle" was a saying I paid little attention to until yesterday. I have been working on finding a fresh way to share the blessing of my Lyme disease experience. This saying really struck a chord for me. It captures the experience in just a few words. To pass through the eye of the needle we have to let go of all we carry with us in life. This was the opportunity of illness for me.

Lyme disease was, without a doubt, one of the best journeys I have ever experienced in my life. It was not enjoyable, it was not fun, and I experienced a wide range of emotions that registered as full on misery. However, as I went through my last year of being sick, I took an introspective look and it was that aspect of the experience that manifested emotions and experiences so profoundly peaceful, forgiving, loving and fulfilling that there simply isn't a spectrum on which to measure them.

After spending the majority of my life participating in athletic endeavors, pursuing interests, work and other activities at the expense of many hours of sleep, it was with immeasurable resistance that I found myself living on the couch under a blanket. All I knew myself to be was stripped away, and I was consumed with guilt and feelings of failure. Hiding from myself in the busyness of life was no longer an option, until I recognized my second line of defense…intellectualizing everything. So from my place on the couch, I put my mind to work. It wasn't long before my cognitive function became severely challenged and thinking, writing and speaking began to falter. My intellect was stripped away too.

With nothing I could do and little I could think, I surrendered, and was left just BE'ing. And in that space of nothingness, free from the baggage of my thoughts, I slipped through the eye of the needle and experienced the richness that is life, the wonder that is my Self, the Oneness that we are, and I learned some lessons.

The letting go of who I knew myself to be allowed me to understand that illness was the perfect expression of my body and mind. Every physiological system expressed itself just as it was, and it was all out of alignment with wellness and well-being. Every ache, pain or malfunction was a signpost for where to look within myself. The illness was not something to avoid or get rid of, it was something to embrace and learn from.

Every day was about nourishing and restoring my immune system with the protocols and diet that resonated with me. My naturopath, chiropractors, energy workers, massage therapists, family and friends were all there to support me to heal within myself. They were wonderful supplements to the primary healing component, Me.

More time was spent exploring and contemplating my thought processes than dealing with the physical aspects of disease. Creating a perspective that was empowering felt so good, and those feelings were the sign posts within which I was finding my alignment. There were many times I wobbled out of alignment, many, but there was simply the return to alignment when I took responsibility for how I had gone out of balance.

Sometimes I look in retrospect at how I've described the healing journey, and sometimes the words have been inadequate. How can one describe the ineffable? But I try anyway and I try here again.
Lyme blessed me with realization:

I realized that I am not, and have never been, broken. Who I am is whole and complete, and this is being expressed into this time/space reality through a physical form.

I realized that who I am is not, and never will be, who I think I am. The mind cannot comprehend the vastness of infinite wisdom and consciousness that I am.

I realized that who I am is who we all are, and what a wonder to experience others through that realization!

I realized that LOVE IS, and that everything is either an expression of love or a cry for love.

I realized that all of life is a blessing, and in aligning with that perspective, it changes the experience of all things I have deemed as negative.

I realized that to wake up to who we truly are requires no knowledge or particular practice or teacher (although they are all helpful). It is simply allowing that which we are to be expressed.

'Knowing' these things does not take away from the human experience, the challenges that life provides, or the contrasting emotional experiences. But 'knowing' from the heart makes it easier to be the observer, easier to step back and look for where I am out of alignment and to expand into broader awareness. My life is my own creation.

For anyone dealing with chronic illness, I would say this;

Here is your perfect opportunity to stop resisting by being present to the moment of now.
Don't resist the experience of your illness, simply allow it. Pushing against your illness puts all your attention on what you don't want, holding you hostage to the problem. In surrendering to what's so in the moment, you will free yourself to attract an experience other than your illness. As an example, if you have ten dollars in your bank account and it's an unwanted balance, and you would rather have $100, thinking only about the ten dollars has you focused on the problem, not the solution.

When you surrender or accept that what you have is ten dollars and you make peace with it, you can then turn your attention to finding a solution that would provide the other $90.

Let go of the thoughts that bring guilt, disappointment and sadness.
They provide nothing other than continued suffering. You

are not wrong or at fault for being ill, you are simply ill.

Create a healing and loving context around every protocol you follow.
Generate thoughts that are authentically self-nourishing. For every bite of food you take or every pill you swallow, imagine the nutrients being transported to all the cells in your body, and 'see' the cells are using them to restore the integrity of your immune system. Each time you detox, visualize the toxins being released from your body, relieving the burden on your body's detoxing systems and organs, and creating efficiency in your internal functions.

Be still; stop trying to figure everything out.
In stillness you will have access to the peace and love that is the essence of your being. Notice how it feels to be still and ask yourself "Who is aware of the feelings?" Be present to this awareness, be the awareness, and you will experience that which is untouched by circumstances and vast beyond the comprehension of your mind, and it is a perfect sense of well-being. It is a journey to be savored for the riches.

After healing through her Lyme experience, Jenny Rush has given up her web site development practice to support others dealing with chronic illness. Never would I have thought that such a deep experience of struggle could have left me with a new purpose and meaning in my life, or leaving me with a new way to be of service to others that is completely fulfilling.

Dennis and Jenny live in Connecticut, and are the parents of two beautiful, grown daughters. They enjoy whatever visiting time they have with them and spend as much time as they can in their house in Maine, a place where they embrace a quiet and simple way of living with their two dogs (the kids that won't leave home).

www.lymethriving.com/

Jill A.

"Your body is more beat up than a retired football player" or "you are a complete mess" or hearing the repeated word "discharged." "We can't help you." What's a girl to do? Cry, or fight back? Maybe a little of both.

When you are faced with a challenging illness, one that is not black and white, one that both mystifies and frustrates some, one that can be personally grueling and unrelenting; how do you cope? Well, put on your big girl panties and join me for a stroll.

Find the support you need.
Words can be hurtful and powerful. Off-the-cuff or negative comments like the ones I mentioned rarely help us in the healing process. We need hope and support and most of all, belief. If a practitioner stops believing in you, Run, Forrest Run! Yes, there are some hard truths, however there is also a lot to uncover about how bodies heal, and every body is different. There are some wonderful, attentive, positive practitioners out there.

Get curious and creative.
I am an admitted treatment Junkie. You name it, I have tried it. Some with success and some without. Be willing to think outside the box, and take reasonable leaps. Over 20 years ago, I tried a little known procedure called Prolotherapy (injections to rebuild the tissue in my body due to systemic joint laxity). I took a chance and it helped me greatly at the time. In fact, it got me back to work for several years.

Subsequent treatments didn't hold, but it certainly bought me some time and there are always new things on the horizon. In fact, I am currently trying energy psychology which utilizes techniques such as Emotional Freedom Technique (EFT or "tapping") to help with my pain and to remove any emotional blocks that may be contributing to my discomfort. Keep in mind, If something isn't working in a reasonable amount of time, it wasn't your thing. Let it go!

Allow versus force.
Allow healing to unfold. It's an unraveling, of sorts, especially if you have been feeling unwell for a while. Force causes stress in the mind and in your body - the very thing you are trying to heal. Think of something you have tried to force in your life; a relationship, a conversation, a treatment perhaps. How did that work for you? Tune in the next time you force something and see how it feels in your body. Then, tune into something wonderful that came into your life when you were in an open and allowing place. Let it unfold!

Preserve your energy.
You will need it to heal. Getting healthy can feel like a full-time job with few benefits. There are a lot of moving parts such as managing your medical records, communicating with and connecting providers, getting to doctors appointments, meeting family obligations and responsibilities. Just making it through the day can feel like a marathon. Choose how you want to spend your time and energy. Who drains you and who lifts you? How can you bring more relaxation into your life? What are you willing or needing to let go of? How can you lighten the load? Answering these questions will help

you get started.

Maintain a sense of humor.
Find the funny or be the funny. Laughing frees us. Know
when you are taking things or yourself too seriously and
snap out of it. Or rap it and YouTube if that lights you up.
When one surgeon I consulted with said "I could pop out
each side of your back in 20 minutes," my reply was "Dude,
this isn't Jiffy Lube, take all the time you need." My Mom,
who was with me at the time gave me that "Honey, don't be
rude look" and then we all, dude included, started laughing.
It was 8:00 p.m., after a four hour consult, out-of-state. We
were all punchy by then and it seemed to free us all.

Be kind to yourself.
I have found that when I get angry with my body, berate it
and dislike what's happening to it, it only inflames things
mentally and physically. Practice self-compassion. Accept
where you are in the moment. It's ok to get frustrated and
wish things were different, because that is natural. Don't
attach to it though. That attachment causes suffering. Your
body drinks in kindness in ways you never could imagine.
Treat yourself with kid gloves.

Keep hope alive.
The answers you want may not be here now, or
tomorrow…remain patient. Don't limit healing to a time
frame or certain way. That will keep you boxed in. Stay
open. Stay curious. You are unique. What didn't work for
one person may work fabulously for you. Rapid changes are
occurring in our medical science and technology and in the

complimentary healing fields. Stay resilient!

What has served me best in my journey is being my own best advocate, seeking the support I wish for, building bridges instead of roadblocks and honoring myself and my unfolding. When I clear the mental chatter and busyness and find ways to bring energy and joy back into my life, I feel like I am living - not simply managing. Keeping my big-girl panties by the way!

Stay present and curious. Be nice to you (others will benefit from this too) and keep hope alive. I wish you all well.

Jill A. is The Little Engine That Could. She is spunky, a little fiery and determined. When she finds herself taking life too seriously, silliness and levity often pull her through. She has learned that resilience often trumps positivity, especially when positivity feels forced. She's mad about football, Thai food, and cats. Jill sometimes takes life more seriously than the situation calls for and when she settles down, she usually can laugh at her bad-ass self. She is Grateful for life's simple pleasures and fun surprises. Jill holds an undergraduate degree in Communications and Health, and a Masters Degree in Organizational Behavior. She also received a Certificate of Completion in Integrative Health Coaching from Duke.

Shawn

Over eight years ago, my journey of healing and transformation began with symptoms of extreme exhaustion and unbearable pain. In addition, I was experiencing uncontrollably heavy, dangerous and publicly embarrassing menstrual bleeding for weeks on end. After many frustrating misdiagnoses and finally the relief of receiving an accurate diagnosis, I was told that the only treatment was major surgery with potentially long-lasting side effects and no guarantee that, at my premenopausal age, the fibroids would not return prior to menopause. I couldn't believe that with such advances in medicine, less extreme options weren't available, but physicians wouldn't budge with their recommendations. And so my research began.

After returning to physicians with alternative healing methods and protocols which had shown to be successful with other women, each physician impatiently dismissed my research as "hogwash", "New-Agey", ineffective and unproven. I was surprised and disheartened that those whom I considered healers were not interested in partnering with me to find a solution that best fit their patient. I quickly learned that I had to be my own health advocate. (I've also since learned that the health needs and issues of women are greatly lagging in medical research.) Luckily, my resolve kicked in to full gear and the next stage of my journey began.

Over the next eight years, fueled by curiosity and fierce determination, I searched to discover not only the true physical and emotional sources of my fibroids, but also healthier and more efficacious treatments that would significantly shrink or even eliminate my fibroids. I worked so very hard. I experimented with many healing methods, herbs and supplements, and every diet I could find. I read book after book and article after article, searched the Web far and wide, and sought treatments from so many alternative health practitioners, only to find temporary relief at best. I couldn't solve the puzzle. I couldn't decipher the messages my body was trying to communicate and the symptoms continued to prevent me from living a normal life. I was beginning to believe those physicians who rolled their eyes at me and lost hope. I was a failure. I had let myself down. I'd hit the lowest and most difficult point of my long journey and I was done. Or so I'd thought.

Feeling so exhausted, defeated and desperate and just wanting my life back, I was ready to finally surrender to the most extreme surgical option of a hysterectomy, regardless of any negative side effects. However, in a serendipitous moment, I wandered into a tiny local bookstore and was drawn to a book that changed my life. Amy Scher had lived the journey and through her book, This is How I Save My Life, I saw that she had truly lived and understood mine. Here was a person who refused to give up and successfully battled through an even more challenging healing journey. One small glimpse of hope had been restored. Maybe someone above was watching over me after all.

I immediately connected with Amy and through my time with her, I was finally shown the gifts of a true and successful healing partnership - endless patience, sensitivity, inspiration, guidance, wisdom, insight to and the healing of unhealthy patterns and beliefs, healing tools, support, compassion, flexibility and encouragement. Through a combination of herbs, supplements, diet and Amy's partnership, tools and therapies, my symptoms significantly subsided and my fibroids shrank in size. It was then when I realized that I had gotten my life back and so much more. What I had gained was truly far more powerful and life changing than the physical healing.

What I have learned from my adventure is that the journey can be long, grueling, and lonely and filled with challenges and setbacks. But if you stick with it, even partner with it, it can be a wise and powerful teacher and spiritual guide. The emotional and spiritual growth is, in fact, far more powerful than the physical healing for the very reason that through the healing process we experience the greater growth of our soul. Along the way, we learn to open our hearts to ourselves. We learn how to love, care for and be a champion for ourselves. We gain a greater understanding of who we are, where we've come from, and who we can be. Choosing to see illness with this perspective helps to give life greater meaning, along with the support needed to return to health.

Additionally, it is really important to keep in mind that every individual is different and no two healing paths and treatment plans are the same. In each moment, trust yourself, be open, experiment and choose who and what feels right for you. And remind yourself that every step you take on your own path, often forward and backward, is wisdom gained and such an inspiring achievement.

Remember to celebrate yourself often. It takes time and patience, so grace and compassion will be asked of you, but you are worth giving it everything you've got. Never give up on yourself. Someone is always watching over you.

Shawn is an energy coach, change agent, spiritual catalyst, writer and leader. She is driven by her passion to inspire, empower and partner with others on their healing journey. www.empowerdigm.com

Alii Goedecke

What was your *One Fun Thing* today…that something special that made you smile? It's a hard question to answer when you're dealing with a chronic illness. But, it may just be the most important question you can ask yourself each day.

It can be unbelievably frustrating and exasperating going through a chronic illness such as Lyme disease. Not understanding the disease for myself, not being able to explain it to others, and not having a standard protocol to follow for wellness were all very frustrating for me.

I had to learn patience and sometimes how to just "let it be." That is where my One Fun Thing each day became a lifesaver for me. Even on the worst of days, with intolerable symptoms, I made sure to find a One Fun Thing in my day. It was my way of keeping control of something good in my life each day. Focusing my energy into a positive place and maintaining a positive attitude kept me hopeful and strong in order to take on each challenge as it came along.

The silver lining in being sick was realizing the importance of One Fun Thing. It resonated with me so strongly that it has become my passion to share that positive message and encourage others to find their One Fun Thing each day.

Whether you are sick or healthy, One Fun Thing is something that can enhance your everyday life. Sometimes it's the small things that make the biggest difference. Your

One Fun Thing can be as simple as calling a friend (might be their One Fun Thing, too!), breathing in the sea breeze or painting your toenails a fun color. It can be anything that brings a smile to your face.

I was grateful to develop this One Fun Thing idea into a children's book as the perfect means to share the idea with others. After all, one of the best things we can teach our children is to have a positive attitude because all great things begin there. Your One Fun Thing can add smiles, fun and energy to any situation.

A highlight of my experience as an author has been hearing how One Fun Thing has touched others' lives. It can be by sharing their One Fun Things around the dinner table each night, or doing a One Fun Thing each day to help bring a smile to their sick child's face. That is an unexpected reward that fills my heart with a feeling of abundance. A perk of where my path has taken me all because of a nasty Lyme bacteria.

We must embrace our journey and become one with it. Be present and experience it fully. As I tell my children, "Don't just go through life, LIVE it!" I may not have had a choice on having Lyme disease, but I made a choice everyday on the attitude by which I lived my life. Finding my One Fun Thing each day was an encouraging way for me to stay focused and present.

People often speak of the silver linings that result from life altering events and I have experienced that firsthand. I found my passion for the message of One Fun Thing that resonated with the essence of who I am. I am thrilled to have had the opportunity to influence others to look at life through that same optimistic viewpoint. I've also been inspired by others' influential ideas: Emotional Freedom Technique (EFT), personalized whole health medicine, affirmations and energy medicine, just to name a few favorites.

It was challenging going through an illness that was so lengthy and so unknown, but taking it one day at a time and finding my One Fun Thing to make me smile each day was a gift. Keep your eyes wide open on your journey because it's astonishing how much you will see, learn and experience. Challenges may come along, whether you like it or not. So, take a moment to enjoy the One Fun Things that come along on your own unique, remarkable journey called Life.

Alii Goedecke lives in Southern California with her husband and two kids who fill her life with One Fun Things! She was inspired to write One Fun Thing while recovering from an extended illness during college. After a two-year medical leave, Alii went on to graduate Phi Beta Kappa, earn an M.B.A. degree and study post-grad at Oxford University and the UCLA's Writers' Program. She has recently recovered from a second bout of chronic illness, which was finally diagnosed and treated as Lyme disease, and looks forward to a bright and healthy future!

*Alii feels that a positive attitude is the best lesson to teach our children because all great things begin there!*One Fun

Thing is a trademark of Alii Goedecke, used with permission for this publication.
www.oneFUNthing.com

Jo

Day 40 (story shared from Jo's blog)
There will be a time, not so far from now, which you will
look back on this phase of your life and instead of
condemning it or beating up on it... Instead of blaming or
guilting, you will feel appreciation for it, because you will
understand that a renewed desire for life was born out of this
time period that will bring you to physical heights that you
could not have achieved without the contrast that gave birth
to this desire. -- Abraham

It's already happened!

In the middle of a busy night, I realized I am grateful to this
illness; truly grateful. If I didn't have it, I would still be
frenetically doing. Now, I have absolutely defined what I
don't want and can get on with designing what I do want.
"As Abraham says, everything is vibrational, and my
thoughts are too, as is illness. So if I eliminate all but the
highest vibrations I must return to Source. And Source is
pure love. No illness." This process doesn't require hours
with a psychologist, just constant monitoring of how you are
feeling emotionally. "Thoughts create emotions, so we have
to choose what we think. If I'm feeling lousy, I'm thinking
something lousy. I have to consciously choose to feel good.

It feels as if I can do this without input from others – a bit
scary to have no limiting factors other than my own beliefs.
I'll take it slowly. Most important is to know I don't have to
be sick or hurt myself to get what I want. I refuse to accept

what I don't want.

"Renewed desire for life" is definitely born. Many times in the past I have longed for death, to re-emerge into the non-physical. I've laid on my bed feeling awful and tried to croak, not knowing how to do it, clearly. I've thought of pills, because I'm no hero when it comes to pain. I believe euthanasia is legal in Holland, and some other places, and have discussed it with Pete. But it seems so limp somehow, to give up. Once a beloved friend begged me for enough pills to end it, and I agonized for weeks. He said the end in his condition was very bad and he just wanted choices. Eventually, I went to my GP and explained the situation and was given a prescription. He was pathetically grateful and slipped the box under his mattress. I don't think he ever used the pills because he died after a long spell in a hospital many years later.

What I also realize is that the reality seems to turn out better than imagined. Somehow one develops a coping style, or an understanding. My husband Fanie's empathy for me is from his place of health and strength; imagining it gone. I've been accepting it bit by bit, working with it, for four years now. It's not pleasant and not what I would choose, but on some level I did choose it and along with it came the grace and ability to handle it. And how lucky I am to have something without much pain.

Am I too old to design a new life? What more important or wonderful to do at 76? Even if I croak in the middle of it, so what. Nothing is ever complete, anyway.

I love synchronicity. Just did Day 11 of Deepak Chopra's 14-Day Meditation Challenge and this was the objective:

"Who am I?" "What do I want?" These two questions may seem simple, but they can be very difficult to answer because they are influenced by the perceptions, wishes and desires of those around you. Once you drop the self-image that has been defined by others, and become more aware of your true self, it will become easier and easier.

Today you will learn a meditation that will help you find your answers to "Who am I?" and "What do I want?" As you begin to accept yourself, you will discover that you do deserve to be happy and content.

I resonated with "self image defined by others" and intend to clarify that. One thing came up that I want for me – apart from the usual abundance, health, love and laughter – is to share what I have learned so that joy and happiness can expand. I haven't a clue how to do that, so need to ask for help and input. I guess being some kind of guide or teacher has always appealed to me as I look at the two books I wrote, as well as the Smokenders (a successful smoking cessation program that addresses the psychological aspects of smoking) classes I taught, and the many SCIO vibrational healing sessions I did (SCIO is a computer-driven biofeedback device that makes over 10,000 frequency readings, from an individual, recording imbalances in every system of the body.

Imbalances, the cause of illness, are then regulated with a combination of 250 individual programs including acupuncture, homeopathy, Reiki, NLP, aura balancing and spinal alignment. Is it arrogant to think I might teach? Is the new me arrogant? Mother voice says, "Don't be so selfish, think of others, not always about yourself."

Answer: if it feels right, then it is right. The Universe will soon give you feedback if it's not right for you. I help no one by being unhappy. I can't expect anybody else to make me happy so that's my main job. Right?

Jo is a 76-year old woman, a lifetime "doer" who was forced into "being" by Parkinson's and Lyme. Jo ordered Amy's book, loved it, and was inspired to write a blog about her recovery. "It is a frank, day-to-day diary of how I wrestle my mind to the mat, to search-and-destroy any limiting or negative thought or emotion. Born in London and raised in America, Canada and South Africa with five siblings, Jo went to 24 schools and worked in public relations, journalism, corporate identity, marketing, property and "green" chemistry. She lives in Johannesburg with her husband Fanie and has a son and daughter. Amy read her blog and said it made her cry. "That's a sign that they touched her truth," says Jo.
www.myrecoveryfromparkinsonsandlyme.blogspot.com

Stacy Shuman

It was one year after my second child was born, 1999, when I began experiencing tachycardia and chest pain. I had my first ride in an ambulance when my youngest was less than two years old. A series of tests with the cardiology department were inconclusive. In the subsequent ten years, I suffered immeasurably with various conditions. My gallbladder was removed, I had an emergency hysterectomy, and on a few occasions I experienced temporary loss of vision. After a significant stress in my life, I developed what we though was the flu, only it came back repeatedly every three weeks for about four months. After the last bout, it disappeared but left in its wake unspeakable fatigue, low-grade fevers and more problems with food. Within two years, I was nearly disabled and my list of symptoms had quadrupled.

With chronic illness, you must first be with your own pain and suffering. When your compassion moves beyond your own condition, you see the pain of others. That has been the most difficult aspect for me. Being awake to the suffering of others, however, can inspire a path of purposeful living. Living with purpose occurs organically when you realize your work and passions have aligned with your highest self, it is about finding your soul work, which can be anything. That is the gift that comes from doing your soul work.

Being ill means being with your "stuff." There is freedom when you can do this honestly because it transitions easily into recognizing that others, for all their awkwardness and fragility, are also dealing with their own "stuff" too. There is so much suffering in the world. When you can relate to that suffering, you instantly feel a part of the world again. When you are in a body that is seemingly failing and without any help or direction from doctors, which happens to many with complex illnesses, there is literally no place to go but "inside."

There is an opportunity when facing extraordinary challenges to create tools for coping. Some of the tools that have worked for me are energy work, breath work, and having a spiritual practice. I love plant-based medicine and aromatherapy. Intuitively, I have always been drawn to nature for healing. For those that are aligned with plant-based or energetic medicine, I would recommend considering this adjunct in your healing protocol. Most holistic doctors I find are very open and positive about this modality. It can be used in so many ways (detoxification, organ support, emotional support, biofilm support, antimicrobial support, etc.,) and it is effective (there are many studies to prove this) and, for the most part, extremely gentle (provided it is used correctly). One of my favorite things to do is to work with the emotional blends during times of detoxification, or where there is Herxheimer response. This is a good time to be extra sweet with your body!

Having a spiritual practice is the singular aspect that has most affected my ability to live with some peace in the midst of pain, fear and uncertainty. People with chronic and complex illness know this; you will fight daily to save your life and with some ambiguity. It can feel impossibly hard, even with support. This is where it helps to believe in something bigger. I had to be completely deconstructed and humbled before it happened to me, but it did happen, and I am grateful beyond measure for it.

I also love using breath work for a few reasons. One, our bodies need oxygen to move our lymphatic's and breathing is the one thing you absolutely can do even if you are bedridden. Two, connecting with your breath is connecting with your body and pain; physical and emotional. That is courageous under the best of circumstances, but it takes monumental courage to do that when the last thing you want to do is be present to your suffering. But it is also powerful to own your suffering and, in my opinion, supports healing. Three, anyone can do this anywhere. I suggest searching on the Internet for ideas to support your breath work practice.

I also love tapping (EFT or Emotional Freedom Technique) for some of the same reasons as I love breath work. It is accessible, affordable, easy and effective. Some of my most powerful shifts occurred when working with a practitioner on this, but you can easily do this work from home.
There is fine line between allowing yourself to be supported by a community and owning your disease. Be mindful about the labels. I am part of the Lyme community, but I still get to decide how I am being defined by this experience. I choose language that is empowering, not leading with my lab reports or symptoms, and finding those in the community that are of like mind.

Stacy Shuman's business venture, as CEO and Founder of Well Scent, began when life took an unexpected turn. She was diagnosed with Late Stage Lyme Disease in 2010. Stacy's journey back to health influenced every aspect of Well Scent, as she became an ambassador for positivity within the Lyme community. Her personal and spiritual transformation created the direction for her business model, which emphasizes the energetic nature of all things.

Well Scent specializes in proprietary organic essential oil formulations that are uniquely created to benefit the immune, endocrine and nervous systems. The line is supported by many physicians, most notably the respected Dr. Klinghardt, founder of the Klinghardt Academy and the Sophia Health Institute. Besides being the CEO & Founder of Well Scent, Stacy is the very proud mother of two incredibly bright, compassionate and self-reliant children, Chaleigh and Matthew. Stacy is now supporting her daughter's healing. Chaleigh's was also diagnosed with Lyme in the winter of 2013.
www.well-scent.com

Nancy Helgeson

I realized that the extreme fatigue I was experiencing could not be normal. I would wake up from a night's sleep, and standing in the shower I felt like a syringe had been inserted in me and that it had sucked out every once of energy that I could possibly have. I was also having other symptoms of depression, extreme memory loss, and barely being able to move through the day. As one friend put it, it was like "walking through peanut butter."

The most difficult part of the experience was dealing with the frustration of the symptoms and not being able to find a diagnosis or the kind of help that I needed. I finally found an MD who was treating individuals with Chronic Fatigue Syndrome. Was he the best help I could find? No. But, at the time (there is much more research on CFS now), most of western medicine considered all of the symptoms to be "in our head." Those of us suffering with the condition were basically told we would just have to put up with it.

Over the next decade, I tried every alternative and natural health care that I thought might help. I even saw a health practitioner that others told me about, but really had no idea where he came from, which I took to mean that he didn't come from this "planet." Nothing really helped in the long run, and during this time I had started my own business, my husband had just left me, and my life had been turned upside down in so many ways. I was attempting to survive financially and keep my head above water so that I wouldn't drown completely.

The MD I was seeing (paying out of my own pocket with no insurance help) told me that he found that most people who had CFS were Type A people, and that we had to learn how to move out of that kind of "life pace" before we could ever heal.

The most important lesson I learned through this journey was that there was no one, or no process, that was going to do the healing I needed. I learned that I had to "take the bull by the horns" and learn self care. The biggest part of that was slowing down, doing less, and enjoying more of the "simple" or "real" things in life.

There is a way out. And I found there are always life lessons in the process of healing. One thing that I did not do was reach out to others to get support. I handled the situation as though I had to figure out everything on my own. My family of origin was not a family who were supportive and that was just who they were. You have to be vulnerable and let people be available to support and help. I almost felt embarrassed by my conditions, because the virus/disease was one that at the time was not fully recognized as being "real."

When you are suffering, you know that it can't be much more real, but you can end up isolating and feeling very alone. All of this was also part of the lessons that I learned and still need to put into practice. Know that you deserve to be supported and loved during your healing, and must look for ways that you can be open to receive that love and support.

Just writing this has helped me reflect on the power of this journey, and the power that I have as a woman who has lived this. Since going through the process, I am still reflecting and learning. I am also in a business where I also need to be available for other people, and to what their needs are. When I am not at my healthiest, I cannot be available for others. This message is still resonating with me.

Nancy Helgeson is an "artist at heart." As a Board Certified Coach and a Licensed Psychotherapist (LMFT), she has been privileged to work with leaders, career transitioners, teams, couples, and individuals from all walks of life. Her work focuses on utilizing a variety of modalities to bring out the best in individuals or organizations.

Nancy is Founder and senior partner of Collaborative Solutions, a firm specializing in Career and Executive Coaching. For the last 25 years, she has served as a Feedback/ Executive Coach and Facilitator for the Center for Creative Leadership and has worked with national and international managers and leaders in a wide variety of industries. Nancy's career has included roles as a corporate human resources manager, a trainer in human development and career development at UCLA and UCSD, an outplacement counselor, individual and marriage therapist, and a parole agent.

Nancy grew up on a Midwestern farm, grounding her in the ways of nature's creativity. After living in the city her entire adult life, she is now finding that her natural creative, artistic and design soul is demanding attention. Creating

Soul Collage and facilitating SoulCollage® workshops brings that alive.

Anne Longpré

When I was about 18 (I'm now 31), I started to feel dizzy, weak, and have severe digestive issues. Things continued to go downhill until a year ago and it got really bad.

The hardest part for me was the feeling of not being normal. I was unable to get out of the house and enjoy anything. I could not participate in social activities and have fun like everyone else.

There was also the fact that it took 12 years to finally be diagnosed with Lyme disease. Until then, doctors said I was crazy and making everything up. Some friends and family, at times, were also questioning whether this was true or not. It came to a point where I hated myself for being so weak and such a hypochondriac. It affected my self-esteem in a huge way.

The financial aspect also was a big stressor for me. I spent $250,000 so far and $75,000 in the last year!

Lyme was, and continues to be, my greatest teacher and friend! Before becoming sick, I already had a number of unhealthy emotional patterns. I was scared that people around me would leave (including that my two-year-old daughter and husband would stop loving me), and I thought that when people did leave it was my fault. Any unexpected expenses such as owing more income tax than planned would keep me awake at night and I thought that everything had to be planned out or else I would be in danger.

Lyme taught me that all of these are not true! I actually realized that I'm responsible for my own well being and situation. Whatever thought you focus on becomes your reality! I've learned that I'm not as weak as I originally thought. In fact, I know that I'm extremely strong and that I can handle pretty much anything life brings to me! I actually love the person I am now and that is quite an achievement considering where I started from. I have also learned that money is not as important as I thought. All that money spent on my health and I'm still alive. It is when you keep thinking that you don't have enough money that you end up with not having enough! This law of attraction is true for every aspect of your life. If you think that you are not good in your work, chances are you won't be. If you think that you are sick, you will stay sick. If you think you are not lovable, no one will love you. When I don't let negative thoughts take over, things work out much better.

The biggest shifts happened over the last year for me and it is still a work in progress. Instead of seeing this as one more thing I have to think about, I'm excited about finding out what else I'm about to learn about myself!

Trust your intuition.
This is what brought me where I am today.

Be happy with everything that you are doing for your health.
If you can't be thankful for the medication that you are taking and everything else that you are doing, it won't help. Also,

most of us are told that a number of things are bad for us and it is most likely true. However, you have to be satisfied with what you are doing now. Of course you can always do more, eat better, get that expensive treatment, etc., but what you are doing now might be all that you need and you won't know unless you believe it.

Take the time to listen to what your illness is trying to tell you.
You will eventually figure it out, I promise!

Surround yourself with people that make you feel good and perfect the way you are.
It's important to be aware that sometimes it is not other people that are making you feel bad, it is your own perception of the situation and of who you are.

Do not participate in "symptoms contests" with people that have the same illness.
If you feel a need for it, there might be core issues that you need to resolve. The term "lymie" makes my stomach turn. It makes me feel gross and weak. If it makes you feel the same way, avoid it at all costs.

Don't give up, but stop fighting!
Trying to "fight" an illness does not put you in the right state to heal. You need to surrender to the whole experience.

I am so grateful to where I am today. Without this experience I would not be half of the person I am and that I'm becoming. I feel so lucky that I learned all of this at my age and that I will be able to teach it to my kids! I would not trade my life and experience with anyone else.

Anne Longpré is a 31-year-old mother of an amazing little girl named Charlotte and has the chance to be with a very loving and caring dad and husband. My professional background is accounting in the public sector. I love outdoors (yes even if there are ticks - although being aware of Lyme has changed the way I approach it a bit!), baking and cooking Paleo meals and treats, listening to music and traveling! I also did EFT courses and love practicing on myself and friends. I have many ideas and plans that I'm keeping to myself at the moment and would love to share once the right moment presents itself!

Lauren Clyde

I am the mother of a teen boy who also has health challenges because of the fact that I had Late-Stage (or Chronic) Lyme disease when I became pregnant (unbeknownst to me at the time) in 1998.

I am an Environmental Scientist who has always wanted to better the planet we live on. For this reason, I went back to college in my mid-20s to begin a new career in water quality protection. I was five years into my new water quality career and just home from my honeymoon when I became ill with very complex and odd symptoms that the doctors I was seeing at the time could not figure out. My symptoms continued and became more concerning shortly after I gave birth to my son in the spring of 1999. Initially, I was diagnosed with Fibromyalgia and Chronic Fatigue Syndrome, just like many others with Lyme disease have been.

Because of the health challenges my son and I have been facing over the last 15 years, and also because of my interest in the health of the planet and our surrounding environment, I have worked to educate myself on how to best heal the body physically as well as emotionally, and use products that have less effect on the environment. This has become an additional passion of mine and I hope to be working on helping others to heal themselves one day soon. This journey has been amazing even though each day often presents big struggles for our family.

Due to my background in science, I often find myself thinking of the process of healing that I am going through as one large-scale science experiment. I find myself wishing for more hours in the day as I want to absorb the studies and information that is available regarding healing. I am finding that I am becoming more connected to the healing process and I am continually amazed at the different topics related to healing which are continually brought to my attention.

Through my work in water quality, I have also become more interested in toxins in the environment and how they may be affecting humans and wildlife. It can be challenging, at times, to keep up with the latest information on these issues while working to heal myself and my child, keep a household running and work part-time. However, I am determined to learn as much as I can and help to heal my family, as well as hopefully many, many others in the future.

One day soon I plan to a write a book that incorporates all that I have learned regarding the various aspects of healing illness (both chronic and acute dis-ease),so that I can help others. I truly feel this is my 'calling' and I sincerely hope that I can help people to heal, as I know it is possible.

I have become even more determined to do this since losing my mom last year. My quest to accomplish this became even stronger last year when my mother, who was very healthy her whole life, went downhill over a period of approximately a year. She passed away suddenly last summer of a type of undiagnosed Non-Hodgkin's Lymphoma that only strikes one in a million people. I want to help people to prevent these types of acute illnesses, as well as to treat and heal from chronic illness by showing them how to incorporate daily healing activities into their lives in balance with nature. Also, how to deal with past emotional traumas that can stress the body and negatively affect the immune system.

Some of the most important things I have learned thus far are that unresolved emotional issues and environmental (including mold and toxins) exposures, can overload a body. In addition, depending on genetics and other factors, this can lead to food and chemical sensitivities and to a state of 'disease' including chronic and/or acute illness.

If you are currently suffering from chronic illness, it is important to figure out what your current environmental stressors are and if you have any blockages to detoxification. One thing I recommend is looking into the work of Dr. Ritchie Shoemaker MD, who has done an amazing amount of research on the issue of mold exposure and how it affects the health of so many. He has found that approximately 25% of the population is extremely sensitive to biotoxins, which includes mold and mycotoxins. Dr Shoemaker has written books on the subject and has a website available with a great deal of information. He developed a protocol for healing the neuroinflammation and other symptoms caused by these exposures. This step is critical to healing in a large number of us who have worked or lived in buildings with water damage.

Another avenue I have pursued that has helped me a great deal is the discovery of genes that limit my ability to detox effectively. One of these genes is the MTHFR gene which encodes the vitamin-dependent enzyme, methylenetetrahydrofolate reductase. There are many health conditions (or defects) caused by functionally impaired forms of the MTHFR protein. These can be improved through dietary supplementation, including specific forms of folate. Genetic testing can be done to determine if you have an MTHFR genetic mutation or other SNPS (Single Nucleotide Polymorsphisms) that are possibly blocking your ability to effectively detoxify. If your body is having trouble with detoxification, this can often lead to or exacerbate existing health issues. I definitely recommend locating a doctor who is familiar with this type of genetic testing. To begin, look into the work of Dr. Amy Yasko for help in navigating these issues.

Addressing sensitivities to common allergens, including food and environmental triggers, can be very helpful in addressing overall health, as well. In many cases, you can be 'treated' for your sensitivities and or allergies so that you can begin to enjoy a specific food or not to react severely to an environmental exposure (such as pollen or grass) again once your body has addressed the sensitivity or allergy. I have had success in utilizing many types of treatment including NAET®, which stands for Namburipad's Allergy Elimination Techniques. NAET is a non-invasive, drug free solution to alleviate allergies and sensitivities using a blend of selective energy balancing, testing and treatment procedures. It uses acupuncture/acupressure, allopathy, chiropractic, nutritional, and kinesiological disciplines of medicine. I also have had success and know many others who have been successful in using other types of similar testing and treatments including; Zyto ™and Autonomic Response Testing (ART) developed by Dietrich Klinghardt, MD, PhD and Lousia Williams, DC, ND. No matter what type of testing or treatment you decide to use, it is important to find a practitioner that has a great deal of experience with the treatment that you choose and one that comes with good referrals from past clientele.

I have also found that using acupuncture and energy healing practices (for example, Reiki or Kairos therapy) can be very helpful in healing both the body and mind. When my mother died suddenly from undiagnosed cancer, I was under an extreme amount of stress and was also told I was in shock following her death. A local energy therapist helped me to release a great deal of the negative emotions and blockages that were associated with this sudden stress and grief in my life. These types of therapies can be very helpful in healing the mind and body, during a particularly difficult period or at any time in life. I have also found that practicing EFT (Emotional Freedom Technique) or 'tapping' is another way to release and resolve negative thoughts and emotions from one's life to allow full healing of the mind and body to occur.

The book I plan to write will address many specific tasks people can implement on their own to improve their overall health, as well as to help prevent and/or heal chronic illness. Some of these practices include minimizing exposure to chemicals in your life by eating a mostly organic diet and using non-toxic personal care and cleaning products. We are exposed to many chemicals daily, without being aware of it in most cases, and limiting our use of household and body care products that contain toxins can greatly reduce daily exposure. Using a filtration system for your drinking water and making sure to drink several glasses of water a day is something I highly recommend. Many cleaning products can be made inexpensively at home using common ingredients including vinegar, baking soda and hydrogen peroxide.

Something that has been very helpful for me and for others I know includes adding simple detoxification procedures to your daily or weekly routine; include taking regular Epsom salt and baking soda baths, dry skin brushing, rebounding, and the use of salt and oil scrubs. One that is particularly simple and effective is making your own salt scrub that can be used in the shower and made easily at home. Salt scrubs help your lymph system to flow properly, which is necessary for good health. They also improve circulation and naturally exfoliate your skin.

Fill a glass jar nearly full with your favorite type of oil (I recommend sesame or safflower) and add sea salt or Epsom salts. If you like, you can add a few drops of your favorite essential oils. Starting at your feet, and moving in the direction of your heart, scrub in a circulatory motion up to your neck. Use this scrub a few times a week in your shower to help your lymphatic system to detox your body. Another important thing you can do to improve overall health is to heal the digestive system. Your overall health starts with this system as it is the foundation of your immune system. Unfortunately, many babies today are not provided with beneficial microflora when they are born as their mothers do not have it to pass along to their child. If you suffer from any digestive issues at all, one of the first things to do is begin taking one or two high-quality probiotics each day. Reducing or preferably completely eliminating sugar from your diet is incredibly helpful and will improve your immune system function as well. Later, when your digestive system is working more effectively, you can add healthy items such as kefir and fermented products such as kombucha. Eating these fermented products regularly is helpful in healing a 'leaky gut' which is very common today and can be very detrimental to overall health. The "Body Ecology Diet" and the "GAPS Diet" are good places to start when looking to heal your digestive system.

I also recommend adding exercises that are healing to your body and strengthen your nervous system. These include yoga or chi-gung and meditation. Meditation is something that is fairly easy to add slowly to your daily routine and it adds huge benefits to your health. Some of the proven benefits you will experience are reduced stress, improved immune function, lowered blood pressure and inflammation. You can begin with as little as just 5 minutes before bed by simply focusing and becoming more aware on your breath. Follow these easy steps to begin your practice:

Sit comfortably. Tune into your breath, follow the sensation of inhaling from your nose to abdomen and out again. Let tension go with each exhalation. When you notice your mind wandering, return to your breath and gently let the distraction go.

Mantra repetition and guided imagery are other types of medication that you can begin to look into and consider adding to your practice. I suggest meditation twice a day for ten minutes at a minimum; however any time at all spent in meditation is worthwhile and has been found to greatly improve sleep..

One day I would like to open a healing clinic offering various forms of healing therapies, such as sauna treatments, massage and energy therapy, and alternative allergy testing, among other treatments, to effectively assist healing and guiding treatments for those that are challenged by chronic and acute illness.

Lauren was diagnosed with Late-Stage Lyme Disease in her late 30's after suffering from a long list of unusual symptoms for over 12 years. She holds a Bachelor's degree in Environmental Studies with emphasis in hazardous materials and water quality. She has always wanted to better the planet we live on as her parents encouraged her to spend time in nature as a child. She hopes to be helping others heal themselves one day soon.
www.facebook.com/lymegreenandhealthyclean

Regina Magee

I am a 43-year-old female and the first sign that something was wrong with my health was when I was 12 years old. It was a long journey, but after 25 years, I was finally diagnosed at the age of 37 with Lyme disease and numerous other tick borne infections, commonly referred to as co-infections.

As if dealing with many health issues wasn't difficult enough, the loneliness of being ill was probably the worst part. In addition, others did not seem to understand the severity of my illness.

According to them, I didn't look sick. It was very hard to feel invalidated by friends and family alike. It often felt like they just didn't believe me. When you can't do what you used to and you have difficulty keeping commitments, you learn quickly who really gets it.

When I first learned that I had Lyme disease, I was very angry. It wasn't so much as "Why me?" as much as I was angry that I felt like I wasn't leading the life I was meant to live. The anger set in just before my diagnosis when I lost my job because I was missing a lot of work. That was a hard pill to swallow. My entire identity was wrapped up in my career and now my career was gone.

Today, I know that what I do for a living has no bearing on my self-worth.

Having said that, being sick has been a blessing in disguise. When you are basically bed-ridden for several years, it gives you a lot of time to think. This experience set me on a spiritual journey that has transformed my thinking in ways that I never thought possible. For example, I was severely depressed from about the age of 13 up until about age 40. I have not been depressed for one single day in the last three years and I no longer wonder what it would be like if I wasn't alive. Now, I wonder what is in store for my future. I know that I am here for a reason. That's not to say that I haven't had the occasional bad day, but I'm not depressed. When those bad moments arise, I now have the tools to turn things around quickly. These past three years have been the most enlightening years of my life in terms of spiritual understanding and personal growth. And for that, I am grateful.

I think there are a few things that someone who has just learned that they have a chronic illness should do for themselves.

Be your own best advocate.
This involves doing research on your illness and finding the right doctors. Not all doctors are alike. If you are seeing a doctor that you feel is not working for you, find another. Do not hesitate to switch doctors.

Find support.
I've heard lots of people say that they feel abandoned by family and friends, but there are many others dealing with what you are dealing with. There are many online and local support groups out there. Look for them and you will find them.

Don't underestimate the power of healing your mind and soul.

We can hold emotional trauma in our body, but it will not heal with traditional medicine. Some ways that this can be done is through prayer, meditation, and other forms of energy healing work such as EFT (Emotional Freedom Technique), Reiki, or IET (Integrated Energy Therapy). This is just a small sampling of the type of energy work available. Follow your intuition and do what you feel is best for you. Remember, we have to be our own best advocates.

Healing my emotional trauma is something that I didn't take into consideration at first. When I finally made the connection between mind, body and soul, that's when I saw a major shift in my health. I've worked on my emotional healing in a few ways. The first is that I've become a Reiki practitioner. By doing this, I can give myself Reiki whenever needed. Reiki is helping me to remove energetic blocks to help promote healing. I've also started doing meditation on a regular basis.

The most profound thing that I've done to heal both emotionally and physically is something called, Advanced Cell Training (ACT). ACT is a unique process that you can do from home. I can't say enough good things about ACT. The gentleman that developed this process is a true healer and he genuinely cares about others getting well.

Everyone dealing with chronic illness should know that things can get better if you believe they will get better. Believing in something, in my opinion, is the most powerful way to create change in your life. Everyone's journey is different, but we are all on a journey nonetheless. Follow your heart and you will get there.

Regina Magee is an Eminent Reiki II Practitioner, working towards becoming an Eminent Reiki Master. She is passionate about all things related to spirituality and energetic healing. She specializes in Distance Reiki so that others can receive healing no matter where they are. www.TheReikiDivas.com

Candice Mitchell

As "they" say, hindsight is 20/20. Looking back at my journey through an enlightened lens, I can now see the signs of the beginning of health issues and warrants for concern, but as a teenager I completely missed the clues. Much like the average American teen, I was consumed with schoolwork, sports teams, social events, college applications, football games and school dances. Any time it felt like my body wasn't working up to par, I brushed it under the rug or made up an excuse for feeling less-than-fantastic. I try to forgive my teenage self for having pretty upside down priorities; chronic illness doesn't come with a handbook. Being an undiagnosed teenager, I didn't exactly have a guide on how to physically, emotionally or socially handle the presence of what seemed like odd symptoms and ailments. Generally, being a teenager is odd enough.

It wasn't until the summer before my junior year in high school that my body began to really struggle and started to shout at me, and despite listening and taking a number of unfruitful trips to a handful of doctors, I didn't get much relief. I continued to live with symptoms that slowly grew in intensity, until I landed in the hospital at age 17, with multi-system failure. The doctors scratched their heads as they tried to figure out why on earth a 17 year old girl's body would just...give up. I had autonomic failure, unresponsive digestive organs, extremely elevated liver enzymes, and suffered an episode of atrial fibrillation.

Every morning, I wake up and remind myself of the role that

132

I want to play in this story. Through my journey, I've learned that we have a choice. Despite the context of the story, the setting, the plot, the "crises", the antagonists...we get to choose who we're going to be. I continue to ask myself: "Am I the hero of this story?" It doesn't always feel that way. But, I've decided that I'm not the victim, and I'm not the damsel in distress. So when I tell this part of my story, I choose not to say that I "nearly lost my life during a hospital stay when I was 17." I don't like to talk about what I missed out on, what changed, or what I had to give up. I like to say that "I survived a really tough hospital stay at 17, and came out a different person on the other side."

When I left that hospital room, I didn't leave with much. I still didn't have a diagnosis. I had no treatment plan. There were no answers and no solutions. Those would come later, with their own set of trials and lessons. But what I did have was a newfound sense of courage and motivation. After about the seventh time watching my own blood pressure plummet on a heart rate monitor, I discovered that fear wasn't going to be very useful in the situation. I divorced the emotion right then and there. So I left fear behind in that hospital room, along with the expectations that I had for my experience as a high school student. Exiting the hospital, I knew I had to start letting go of what I thought my life was supposed to look like, and start accepting the responsibility of figuring out how to manage my own health. Clearly, there wasn't going to be a knight in shining armor to do it for me. Not in this story, at least.

After I left the hospital, I did all that I could to support my body and regain my strength. I changed my diet, I went gluten free, and I went back to a holistic physician who helped me put together a protocol that would address some of my symptoms. Committing to alternative medicine and lifestyle changes were what ultimately pulled me through the remainder of my high school years, where I went to school half days and was able to graduate with my class. I even got into University of California, Davis, and had gained enough strength to move out and give attending college a shot.

I made it through two quarters at UC Davis before my body began to protest again. Trying to manage being a college student and an undiagnosed patient was an experience. I'm quite confident in saying that I was probably the only student in my dorm that had a vegetable steamer under her bed, probiotic cocktails in her mini fridge, and rice cake crumbs all over her floor. In the beginning of my third quarter, my symptoms intensified, which oddly manifested in heart rate abnormalities and a largely inflated spleen. Landing in the hospital again didn't sound like an optimal plan, so I came home for assessment and treatment. The gigantic spleen was probably the first clue to my holistic physician that the root of my illness was likely infectious. After a round of tests, I finally received a diagnosis.

I wish I could say that it was "all uphill from there", but that wasn't exactly the case. I do like to think though that it was the beginning of the beginning of the rest of my life. I think of it as my detour to the path that I was always meant to be on, that I know will lead to the place I'm meant to be.

I think that one of the most difficult parts of chronic
learning to let go. It's tough to let go of what you th
your life should have or could have looked like, and it's hard
to release expectations, drafted road maps, and time-
constrained dreams.

One of my favorite quotes that I've come across along the
way has been one by Dr. Rachel Naomi Remen: "Healing
may not be so much about getting better, as about letting go
of everything that isn't you - all of the expectations, all of the
beliefs - and becoming who you are."

Living with chronic illness is often physically painful. But
somewhere along the way, I learned that it doesn't always
have to be an emotionally and spiritually excruciating
experience. I think that a lot of the emotional and spiritual
pain comes from resistance. I think that once you let go of
the "would'ves, should'ves, and could'ves", it frees up space
for joy and peace to come in. Sometimes, even unexpected
opportunity. Once you release the chains of expectation,
you're free to begin to learn and grow.

My most important lesson? Just say no to the cookie.

Unfortunately, your immune system doesn't understand when
you decide that you're "gluten free, except for on Tuesdays."

When I was first beginning on my journey, I wish someone
had told me not to be ashamed. That my diagnosis wasn't my
fault, and that a loss in physical strength didn't mean that I
was weak. I wish someone had told me not to hide. I think

that in our society, we're influenced and cultured to believe that strength and beauty are rooted in physical characteristics. But I feel as though I've been gifted with the chance to view strength and beauty through an alternative lens. Experiencing illness has lead me to meet people and witness things that have demonstrated strength that can't be measured by miles ran or weights lifted, and beauty that can't be washed away with water or time.

So, if there was one piece of advice I'd give someone who was just beginning their journey, it would be to not be ashamed to let people in. Allow them to see you and be with you where you're at. In the absence of physical strength, don't allow shame to seep in and take its place. You are strong. I'm willing to bet that you have more courage and endurance than anyone else around you. You are beautiful. There's nothing more beautiful than someone who can demonstrate optimism and compassion in moments of vulnerability and struggle.

Candice Mitchell has learned over the past seven years that while Lyme disease may be infectious, so is optimism, and we all need a little optimism in order to get by.

Autoimmune and neuroimmune illness is complicated and undoubtedly challenging. But with commitment, courage, patience and a holistic mentality, she believes that it is possible to heal. Candice believes that in order to achieve wellness and maintain health, it's necessary to revisit the basics and get down to earth. Natural healing modalities, as well as food can be medicine. Hope can be found in every bite.

So, please join Candice in a quest for health as PB&J sandwiches are traded in for almond butter and celery, swap out perfume and hair mousse for argan and olive oil, and replace pharmaceuticals with potions and remedies. Every lifestyle change made is a step toward wellness.
And just in case you haven't heard, Candice says "being a late stage Lyme patient automatically makes you a badass."
http://www.infectiouslyoptimistic.com

Jocie Vortman Van Reusen

It's hard to say when I first realized something was off with my health. I have always been incredibly aware of my body and had myriad somatic symptoms starting in grade school. I would say my twenties - after college - was when physical symptoms became overwhelming loud in my life. It didn't seem normal to be having colonoscopies, MRIs, heart monitors and lab work at the rate I did during those years, but I also knew something was seriously wrong with my body and was determined to find out the culprit. Because I had struggled with anxiety most of my life, it was an easy go-to for doctors to explain away the symptoms and most of the time I bought it, which only made things worse for me. I was finally diagnosed with Lyme in 2009, and of course, from there, the testing and doctors and pills and lab work and search and controversy only increased.

The most difficult part of being ill was truly being so lost in the wilderness that I couldn't see out.
Many relationships were lost or injured during those years because I didn't even know which way was up, let alone explain to others what was happening inside of me and why I didn't want to see them or return their phone calls. There was zero clarity at times and I just sank with distress. I didn't know how to help myself and there was too much information to sort through, learn, and conquer.
Of course, it didn't help that there was so much controversy around the disease and very few understood what Lyme disease was - including local doctors - and how it affected so many systems of the body. It took a long time (years) for me

to un-layer the illness developed in my system and w
piece of un-layering and a boatload of support, I event
gained more clarity and could start to direct my treatment
rather than be directed.

There are too many lessons to share! People seem to look at
me funny when I tell them I'm actually grateful for Lyme &
Co. coming along. It's true. As painful as it has been and how
my life was ruled by fear, I see it ultimately as an
opportunity to find true healing from the inside out. Perhaps
the most important revelation along my journey was when I
realized it wasn't about Lyme at all. I distinctly remember
telling one of my most beloved Lyme doctors just that and it
being a profound shift in my healing. It's not that I knew
exactly what it *was* about. I didn't! But, I knew I had become
so identified with being sick, my symptoms, and the search
for health that it didn't matter anymore what drugs, herbs,
homeopathy or treatments I tried. None of it was going to
work, because some part of me didn't want it to work. I was
blocking my own healing without knowing it.

I didn't know who I was or what life would be like without
the illness. I didn't know what it felt like to be symptom free
and the thought scared the crap out of me. It seemed
contradictory since it was my full time job to get well, but I
knew on some level that I had made the journey of healing
about killing Lyme. But, it really was about bringing my
authentic self to life in a way I had never known. I didn't
have boundaries, couldn't say no, avoided all conflict, and
had no idea how to name and express my feelings in a
reasonable way. My energy was jacked, there was crap to

clear, beliefs to bust and a little girl inside who desperately needed my love and to know that it was okay to be her, no matter what that looked like.

I could go on an on, but Lyme for me has been a gift of self-discovery, of finding my wild, and digging in to weed out the junk that wasn't serving me anymore, no matter how attached to it I may have been. The more I dig and the more love I give to myself, my health increases exponentially.

Try not to get caught up in symptom sharing and conference hopping.

My doc called me a conference junkie. It can sometimes be helpful, but can also perpetuate a negative energy that keeps us stuck. Lyme manifests incredibly different in each person, so comparing is for the birds.

See the Lyme not as the enemy, something to be destroyed, but rather as a teacher trying to show you something.

While you are in treatment, continue to ask your body's wisdom to reveal to you what it is that you need to see; what it is that truly needs to be healed in your being. Be open to the feedback you receive and be willing to explore it little by little.

Find a doctor (or practitioner) who resonates with you.

I have had the benefit of a multi-disciplinary team, but my main LLMD was found after several tries with docs that didn't fit with my style. He is casual, doesn't wear a white coat and is brilliantly intuitive and funny. It took me awhile to realize that's why I connected, but my gut told me the second I met him. So, follow your gut! Ultimately, you are your greatest healer, but often times we (as I did) need healers outside of us to show us the way and love us through it. The down side of being well for me is not seeing him! I wish for everyone to have that relationship with their healer.

Get to know how to love and care for yourself deeply and practice it every day.
Also, if you are trying to heal on a budget, there are loads of books out there to read, some of which are at your local library. I felt empowered by learning on my own, even when I couldn't have a one-on-one with Louise Hay. I wish you a bad-ass journey of joy through it all.

Jocie Vortman Van Reusen lives in Southern California with her husband and several beloved pets.
http://www.jociev.com/

Janice Perkins Fairbairn

Last summer, my five-year-old daughter struggled with putting her face in the water during swimming lessons. After a few days, we began to practice the face-in-the-water technique in the bathtub.

Then in swimming lessons, she would get fearful and not even try it at all. So, the next bathtub training session, I began to ask her why she could do it so well at home and not in the pool. She looked at me and simply said, "The pool has a deep end."

Well, that didn't deter me and I continued explaining that she is roped off in the shallow end, far away from the deep end and should have no fears of it. Her irrational simple reply came again, "But I can see the deep end."

As I clamored out of the Valley of the Shadow of Lyme, I realized what the depths of that pit were to me. Enduring this Lyme disease battle is not for the faint of heart. It requires nerves of steel, perseverance and serious "gumption." A soldier built for a battlefield of this kind of terror I am not. I could not only see the "deep end" of my Lyme disease, I was sinking in it.

I had experienced fear like this only once before, the kind that takes your breath away. On 9/11, I was in New York and worked two blocks from the World Trade Center. My commute involved taking the Path train into the subbasement of the WTC each morning. One thing I can tell you though was, when the fighter jets scrambled overhead within minutes, it came like reassurance that someone had my back. I was not down there alone in battle. The army has been called. On alert, the soldiers are on their way. Someone is on this.

In the face of Lyme, I experienced that fear again - absolute terror. As my journey continued though, I found that the "jets scrambled" became my faith, an incredible community of Lyme warriors and the love of friends and family. Someone is on this. We are all in this and on this together. I was not about to sink in my "deep end of the pool."

How did it start for me? Well, I had a miscarriage, two difficult deliveries, early onset perimenopause and borderline glaucoma. Soon after kids, I began to get some more hormone swinging and "anger" that was driving me crazy. Both my kids had severe digestion and behavior issues. My son would have been diagnosed Asperger's and we were losing him farther down the spectrum before we began to do more health changes. My daughter had asthma, speech delays, hearing, emotional and sleep disturbances. My life was a constant duct-taped stress ball. Held barely together at the seams, it felt like the person at the circus trying to keep all the plates spinning in the air. Those plates crashing down became a fear I lived with daily.

Sicker and sicker I became. There was more and more weight loss, no sleep, immense pain in chest, heart and under ribcage. I couldn't drive, couldn't read, and I felt like I was going blind.

I had been diagnosed Sjogren's, Lupus, Hashimoto's, Glaucoma and other possible autoimmune diseases.

After finally receiving a positive for Lyme on a Western Blot, I began three weeks of doxycycline.
At this point I was probably 95 lbs. and very weak and exhausted emotionally and physically. I had already been up and down for almost five months. But we had our answer and it would be over soon. People get this all the time, right? They just take antibiotics and live life. Wrong.

This began the darkest days I have ever experienced and I wouldn't wish upon my worst enemy. What I didn't know at the time was that what I had been experiencing was herxing. Severe herxing. Some that caused us to go the Emergency Room again and again. The worst had me in full body tremors/seizures.

It was at the end of these three weeks that I finally looked at my husband and said call the church and ask for prayer. I just knew I was going to die. Down to below 85 lbs. and unable to eat, and the pain was unbearable.

After the prayers went out, three days in a row by three different people I was handed a Lyme doctor's name. What I didn't know then that I know now was that the neurotoxin and ammonia overload from the Cat's Claw, the ozone, the Colloidal Silver and finally the Doxy had flooded my system in trying to kill off the Lyme and co-infections. I was herxing myself right to the grave. My brain and heart were filled with ammonia, my gall bladder, liver and kidneys were

144

80% non-functioning. My lymph system was a clogged up solidified mess and my blood was not only thick and lifeless, but not flowing out of my brain due to jugular blocks from the Lyme bacteria.

I was as good as dead. In that health condition, I bet I wouldn't have lasted more than a few weeks. God had other plans.

The Lyme doctors I chose do a holistic approach with no antibiotics. They also do not believe in herxing.

I had been in a herx for nearly four weeks straight without a break. The other ones had come in three to ten days waves and usually dissipated a bit. This one had come in to camp and hadn't left. I was so thin that I had to use a butt pillow to sit on most of the chairs in our house.

The doctors there at Hansa Center of Optimum Health, the founder a former Lymie, developed this protocol to save his own life, antibiotic free. They believe in detoxing the ammonia and neurotoxins as a top priority in order to then strengthen your body to fight off the Lyme itself, as it was designed to do.

The oddest thing they told me and it took weeks before I could actually cognitively process the information: that I had a condition called CCSVI.

CCSVI standing for Chronic Cerebrospinal Venous Insufficiency means that the Lyme bacteria has caused closures in the jugular veins coming out of my brain so the blood flowing into the brain has no place to flow out. My left side almost completely closed off and the right side about halfway. So what happens to the blood being pumped into the brain if it has no way out? Well, it causes tremendous pressure and iron buildup in the tissue and flows backward down the arteries. It goes Up-river so to speak. It is called back flowing. It causes erratic heart beats, severe chest pressure and pain, brain fog and memory loss.

After the second month of treatment, it hit me like a tidal wave. "My kids have Lyme" was whispered to the very bottom of my soul and I was certain it was true. That is why they have been struggling since birth. Tests confirmed they had everything I had and we began treatment for them too.

I chose to tell you all this so you know I have walked into the deepest part of the valley where you are or where you have been. I have met people who suffered more and less. I have met three generations in one family all suffering all the way down to the eight year old. I have met entire households struck with this terrible illness and all fighting for their lives. I get passionate; I get fired up at the lack of support from the traditional medical community and how hard you have to fight upriver to get traction in this illness. I get frustrated on how much money it costs to pay all these treatments out of pocket because there is no alternative in traditional medicine. If there was enough money on our money tree, I would give it all to people desperate to get natural treatment but can't afford it. So here I share with you the tips I feel are most helpful:

Get an advocate.
Find someone, in your family, a neighbor, a friend, your spouse or a grown child to be your advocate. Lyme disease saps the brain cells right out of a person and throws you into confusion. Your advocate can go to doctor's appointments with you, do research online, make sure you are taking the right stuff at the right times and even help you organize fundraisers. Ask them to email or blog for you until you can to keep in touch with "life" and what's going on. Feeling left out and missing months or years is a terribly lonely place to be for a Lymie.

Plug into a support group online or in-person.
Get in front of other Lymies, but make sure it is a positive supportive group of people that are healing and helping.

Make friends at the doctor office.
When I began going to a Lyme doctor, I certainly felt like I could barely walk in the door, but I was determined to "make friends" with every Lyme patient I bumped into in the office. I wanted to see who was surviving and thriving and make sure I had come to a place that was healing and succeeding.

Ask for help and accept the help you need.
I am not a person who asks for help, EVER. This disease really stretched me beyond a vulnerability that I had ever experienced before. But I had two little kids at home and couldn't drive or function most days. I had to humbly accept help. First I had to evaluate where I needed help the most and what would benefit my kids and family the best.

147

Be willing to do anything, look anywhere and rebuild your foundation of health beliefs.
Lyme disease is not main stream and there is no sure fire method of healing that works the same for every person. Let this illness and what it's doing to your body guide where you need to go for help and healing.

Strengthen your resolve.
This Lyme battle is not for the faint of heart. It will build character or tear you to pieces. In order to remain strong, you must input into your body, mind and spirit positive information. Read uplifting success stories, a daily devotional, or the bible. Listen to positive uplifting encouraging music or audio books.

Keep finding laughter and a reason for living each day.
Don't give up making plans. Some will happen and most will not, but don't keep trying. The momentum will shift and the percentages will soon be in your favor. If you don't put goals and plans on the calendar, you will have nothing to look forward to or fight for. Fun and laughter are critical for this journey.

Celebrate the small successes along the way.
The Lyme journey does not happen in big giant gains or jumps. It happens more like baby steps and a gradual climb out of the hole. Stop and look back and remember how far you've come; it will give you the courage to keep it up. Practice gratefulness and build a timeline or journal or blog. Remembering from where you've come helps the heart be

more fertile ground for gratefulness.

Prepare for the marathon.
Don't place unreasonable expectations on your doctor or healing journey. Lyme is not a sprint. It is a long haul. Enjoy the journey, though, there will be wonderful moments of surprising health and clarity. Take advantage of those days - those "open windows" of energy and health and get out and do something. Don't listen to people who tell you not to overdo it. You might not know when the next window of opportunity to feel this good will be, so make it great.

Don't put off getting your Lyme degree - knowledge is power.
Lyme is a new illness gaining ground and information and treatments every day. It is imperative that you learn the lingo and figure out how to navigate the minefield of vocabulary and treatments. Use your advocate until you can get your brain cells up to speed again.

My journey and my valley are not over. Our family's battles continue but we have a winning record. We are chipping away at what Lyme has done in our home.

I am driving, I am reading, and I am writing. Most importantly, I am living with my eyes focused forward and upward. Trying to see all wonderful gifts given each day in light of the character building God is doing in our family.

We have come a long way and as I write this, it is a good

reminder to be thankful and continue the fight.

When I look in the mirror now I see a ton of more gray hairs, but I see life. I see my soul reflecting back a life that was worth fighting for and worth keeping.

My goal for myself and my kids is to live life to the full knowing that each breath is a gift from God. For us to use our talents and experiences to help others find hope and healing. In small measure, I pray for continued strength and for cow's cheese to re-enter our house to be devoured in late night snacks. My son's goal is to someday eat Papa John's pizza. Maybe someday we will. But until then, I just found out a new pizza place down the street is serving gluten free pizza...

Janice Perkins Fairbairn discovered she had Lyme over two years ago, simultaneously discovered she had given her two kids everything while they were in the womb. All three of them began a natural form of treatment for Lyme because of intolerance to the antibiotics. She got down to below 85 lbs in her Lyme valley and had to climb out of it and pull her kids out with me. All by the grace of God. She is compelled to share my story and journey to encourage others it can be done. Hold onto hope. She is the author of My God, My Lyme; Surviving Lyme; Support in Lyme for Families and Advocates.
www.justlivinglikethiswithlyme.com

.

About Amy B. Scher

Amy B. Scher is a bestselling author, expert in mind-body-spirit healing, and is often lovingly referred to as an "accidental guru."

Her books and her work have been featured in publications such as CNN, Curve magazine, Divine Caroline, The Tapping Solution, Psych Central, and the San Francisco Book Review. Amy was named one of Advocate's "40 Under 40" for 2013 and has presented to groups including the Department of Psychiatry and Behavioral Sciences at Stanford University, and the Harley-Davidson Motor Company.

As a minister of Holistic Healing, Amy uses energy therapy techniques to help those struggling with emotional or physical challenges to identify, release, and move on.

Most importantly, she lives by the self-created motto: "When life kicks your ass, kick back."

www.amybscher.com

One Last Thing

Become Part of My Family

My life's goal is to help people turn from their 'stuckness' and embrace a better path. If you or someone you love would like my help in shifting your energy to a more balanced place, please visit my website for lots of cool tricks and training: *www.amybscher.com*

One Last Thing…

When you turn this page you'll be greeted with a request from Amazon to rate this book and post your thoughts on FaceBook and Twitter. How cool is that? Your friends get to know what you're reading and I, for one, will be forever grateful to you.

All the best,
Amy